Biochemical

s

This book is to be returned on
or before the date stamped below

UNIVERSITY OF PLYMOUTH

PLYMOUTH LIBRARY
Tel: (0752) 232323
This book is subject to recall if required by another reader
Books may be renewed by phone
CHARGES WILL BE MADE FOR OVERDUE BOOKS

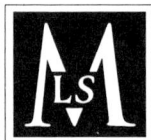

CRC Press
METHODS IN THE LIFE SCIENCES

Gerald D. Fasman - *Advisory Editor*
Brandeis University

Series Overview

Methods in Biochemistry
John Hershey
Department of Biological Chemistry
University of California

Cellular and Molecular Neuropharmacology
Joan M. Lakoski
Department of Pharmacology
Penn State University

Research Methods for Inbred Laboratory Mice
John P. Sundberg
The Jackson Laboratory
Bar Harbor, Maine

Methods in Neuroscience
Sidney A. Simon
Department of Neurobiology
Duke University

Joseph M. Corless
Department of Cell Biology,
Neurobiology and Ophthalmology
Duke University

Methods in Pharmacology
John H. McNeill
Professor and Dean
Faculty of Pharmaceutical Science
The University of British Columbia

Methods in Signal Transduction
Joseph Eichberg, Jr.
Department of Biochemical and Biophysical Sciences
University of Houston

Methods in Toxicology
Edward J. Massaro
Senior Research Scientist
National Health and Environmental Effects Research Laboratory
Research Triangle Park, North Carolina

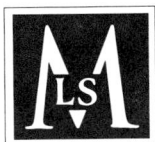

CRC Press
METHODS IN PHARMACOLOGY

John H. McNeill
Faculty of Pharmaceutical Sciences
The University of British Columbia
Vancouver, B.C. CANADA

The *CRC Press Methods in Pharmacology Series* provides the reader with a step-by-step approach to each of the classical and up-to-date methods and presents techniques in a clear and concise format. Topics covering all aspects of pharmacology are being reviewed for publication.

Published Titles

Biochemical Techniques in the Heart, John H. McNeill
Measurement of Cardiac Function, John H. McNeill
Measurement of Cardiovascular Function, John H. McNeill

Forthcoming Titles

Methods in Cardiac Electrophysiology

Biochemical Techniques *in the* Heart

Edited by

John H. McNeill, Ph.D.

Department of Pharmaceutical Sciences
University of British Columbia
Vancouver, Canada

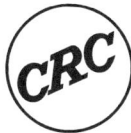

CRC

CRC Press
Boca Raton   New York   London   Tokyo

Senior Acquiring Editor:	Paul Petralia
Editorial Assistant:	Cindy Carelli
Project Editor:	Helen Linna
Direct Marketing Manager:	Becky McEldowney
Marketing Manager:	Susie Carlisle
Cover Design:	Denise Craig
PrePress:	Carlos Esser
Manufacturing:	Sheri Schwartz

Library of Congress Cataloging-in-Publication Data

Biochemical techniques in the heart / edited by John H. McNeill.
     p.   cm. — (CRC Press methods in the life sciences. Methods in pharmacology)
    Includes bibliographical references and index.
    ISBN 0-8493-3333-4
    1. Cardiology, Experimental — Laboratory manuals. 2. Sarcolemma —
-Research — Laboratory manuals. 3. Heart cells — Research — Laboratory
manuals. 4. Cardiovascular pharmacology — Laboratory manuals.
I. McNeill, John H. II. Series.
    [DNLM: 1. Heart — physiology — laboratory manuals. 2. Biochemistry —
-methods — laboratory manuals. WG 25 B615 1996]
QR112.4.B56 1996
612.1'73--dc20
DNLM/DLC
for Library of Congress
                            96-29039
                               CIP

© 1997 by CRC Press, Inc.

No claim to original U.S. Government works
International Standard Book Number 0-8493-3333-4
Library of Congress Card Number 96-29039
Printed in the United States of America 1 2 3 4 5 6 7 8 9 0
Printed on acid-free paper

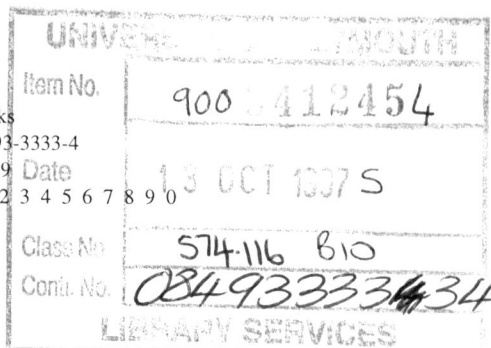

Dedication

To my wife Sharon and my daughters Sandy and Laurie.
You are always there for me.

Preface

The books in this series have been conceived as a trilogy on "Methods in Experimental Cardiology" and represent the only texts providing a detailed description of the main techniques used in understanding physiological and pathophysiological cardiovascular regulation. In order to enhance the effectiveness and readability, the work has been divided into three volumes. Volume 1, *Measurement of Cardiac Function,* includes chapters on The Langendorff Heart, The Isolated Working Heart, Isolated Papillary Muscle Preparations, Isolated Atrial Muscle Preparations, *In Vivo* Measurements of Cardiac Function, and Isolated Ventricle Measurements. Volume 2 is entitled *Measurement of Cardiovascular Function* and includes chapters on The Lipid Perfused Heart, Metabolic Measurements in the Heart, Models of Arrhythmia, Techniques for Arterial Blood Pressure Measurement, and Models of Experimental Hypertension. Volume 3, *Biochemical Techniques in the Heart,* deals with Preparation of SR, Preparation of Sarcolemma, Measurement of Sodium-Calcium Exchange, Measurement of Sodium-Potassium ATPase, Molecular Assessment of the Sodium-Potassium ATPase, Measurement of Sodium-Hydrogen Exchange, and Preparation of Cardiomyocytes.

Each chapter has been peer-reviewed and carefully edited in order to provide an up-to-date, comprehensive, practical, portable, and accessible guide to the main experimental techniques used in examining *in vivo, ex vivo,* and *in vitro* cardiac function in animals. The text answers a long-felt need and represents the contribution of an outstanding group of authors who provide the cardiovascular audience with the *"recipe"* of the techniques: setting up the method, starting materials required and their procurement, the "do's and don'ts," troubleshooting and resolution, sample data, spreadsheets and calculations, and modifications and applicability.

With multiple flowcharts, diagrams, and actual photographs, these simple and straightforward texts will serve both as a research reference and a bench guide for the cardiac physiologist, pharmacologist, biochemist, and trainee and will hopefully save hours of precious research time.

John H. McNeill, Ph.D.
Professor and Dean
Faculty of Pharmaceutical Sciences
The University of British Columbia

The Editor

John H. McNeill, Ph.D., is Professor of Pharmacology and Toxicology and Dean of the Faculty of Pharmaceutical Sciences at The University of British Columbia in Vancouver, Canada.

Dr. McNeill graduated in 1960 from the University of Alberta with a B.Sc., (Pharm) degree. He obtained his M.Sc. from the same institution 2 years later and his Ph.D. in Pharmacology at the University of Michigan in 1967.

Dr. McNeill is a member of the Pharmacological Society of Canada, the American Society for Pharmacology and Experimental Therapeutics, the Western Pharmacology Society, the International Society for Heart Research, the Association of Faculties of Pharmacy, American Pharmaceutical Association, Sigma Xi, American Diabetes Association, Canadian Diabetes Association and Canadian Pharmaceutical Association. Dr. McNeill served on the Council and as President of the Canadian Pharmacology Society and the Western Pharmacology Society and on the Council of the North American Section and the international body of the International Society for Heart Research. He has served on and chaired many Canadian national research committees for the MRC, Canadian Heart and Stroke Foundation, Canadian Diabetes Association, and the PMAC–Health Research Foundation. He currently serves on the jury for the prestigious Prix Galien Award.

Dr. McNeill has received a number of awards for his research including the Upjohn Award (Canadian Pharmacology Society), McNeil Award (Association of Faculties of Pharmacy of Canada), and the Jacob Biely Award and Killam Award from The University of British Columbia. He has been an MRC Visiting Professor at a number of Canadian universities and at Montpellier University in France.

Dr. McNeill has presented numerous invited lectures in North America, Europe and Japan and has published over 350 manuscripts, reviews and book chapters. His current major research interests are diabetes-induced cardiomyopathy, hyperinsulinemia and hypertension, glucose-lowering agents, and mechanisms of action of insulin.

Contributors

Naranjan S. Dhalla, Ph.D., M.D. (Hon.)
Institute of Cardiovascular Sciences
St. Boniface General Hospital
  Research Centre and
  Department of Physiology
Faculty of Medicine
University of Manitoba
Winnipeg, Manitoba, Canada

Vijayan Elimban, Ph.D.
Institute of Cardiovascular Sciences
St. Boniface General Hospital
  Research Centre and
  Department of Physiology
Faculty of Medicine
University of Manitoba
Winnipeg, Manitoba, Canada

Kiminori Kato, Ph.D., M.D.
Institute of Cardiovascular Sciences
St. Boniface General Hospital
  Research Centre and
  Department of Physiology
Faculty of Medicine
University of Manitoba
Winnipeg, Manitoba, Canada

John J. Leddy, Ph.D.
Department of Pharmacology
Faculty of Medicine
University of Ottawa
Ottawa, Ontario, Canada

Anton Lukas, Ph.D.
Institute of Cardiovascular Sciences
St. Boniface General Hospital
  Research Centre and
  Department of Physiology
Faculty of Medicine
University of Manitoba
Winnipeg, Manitoba, Canada

Hamid Massaeli, B.Sc.
Ion Transport Laboratory
Division of Cardiovascular Sciences
St. Boniface General Hospital
  Research Center
Winnipeg, Manitoba, Canada

Grant N. Pierce, Ph.D.
Ion Transport Laboratory
Division of Cardiovascular Sciences
St. Boniface General Hospital
  Research Center
Winnipeg, Manitoba, Canada

Brian Rodrigues, Ph.D.
Division of Pharmacology and
  Toxicology
Faculty of Pharmaceutical Sciences
University of British Columbia
Vancouver, British Columbia, Canada

David Severson, Ph.D.
Department of Pharmacology and
  Therapeutics
Faculty of Medicine
The University of Calgary
Calgary, Alberta, Canada

Glen F. Tibbits, Ph.D.
School of Kinesiology
Simon Fraser University
Burnaby, British Columbia, Canada

Balwant S. Tuana, Ph.D.
Department of Pharmacology
Faculty of Medicine
University of Ottawa
Ottawa, Ontario, Canada

Acknowledgments

I would like to thank Jeff Hillier who first discussed the idea for these books with me many years ago and Paul Petralia who arm-wrestled me into finding the time to actually go ahead and bring the project to fruition. Two of my graduate students, Margaret Cam and Subodh Verma reviewed all of the book chapters from the perspective of a graduate student. Subodh was my strong right arm in badgering authors, helping me edit, and ensuring that everything was done properly. To him, I owe a tremendous debt.

Contents

Chapter 1. Preparation of Cardiac Sarcoplasmic Reticulum 1
John J. Leddy and Balwant S. Tauna

Chapter 2. The Isolation of Myocardial Sarcolemma 17
Glen F. Tibbits

Chapter 3. Measurement of Na^+-Ca^{2+} Exchange 31
Glen F. Tibbits

Chapter 4. Measurement of Sodium/Potassium
ATPase in Myocardium 45
*Vijayan Elimban, Anton Lukas,
and Naranjan S. Dhalla*

Chapter 5. Molecular Assessment of Cardiac
Sodium Pump Activity 63
*Vijayan Elimban, Kiminori Kato,
and Naranjan S. Dhalla*

Chapter 6. Methods for Measuring Sodium-Hydrogen
Exchange in the Heart 83
Hamid Massaeli and Grant N. Pierce

Chapter 7. *Preparation of Cardiomyocetes* 101
Brian Rodrigues and David L. Severson

Index 117

Chapter

1

Preparation of Cardiac Sarcoplasmic Reticulum

John J. Leddy and Balwant S. Tuana

Contents

1. Introduction 2
    1.1. Applications 2
        1.1.1. Ca^{2+} Transport 2
        1.1.2. Protein Purification and Characterization 3
        1.1.3. Electrophysiology 4
    1.2. Overview of Isolation Procedures 4
2. Method for Isolating Cardiac Sarcoplasmic Reticulum 4
    2.1. Preparation of Solutions 5
    2.2. Centrifugation 5
        2.2.1. Differential Centrifugation of Heart Homogenates 6
        2.2.2. Discontinuous Gradient Centrifugation of the Heart
                Membranes 7
    2.3. Determination of Purity 8
        2.3.1. [³H] Ryanodine Binding Assay 8
        2.3.2. Other Sarcoplasmic Reticulum Markers 9
    2.4. Examples of Data Obtained 9
    2.5. Potential Problems 10
3. Summary 12
Acknowledgments 12
References 12

1

1.   Introduction

The cardiac contraction-relaxation cycle is precisely regulated by the level of cytosolic calcium ion. Contraction is initiated when the Ca^{2+} level reaches a threshold of binding to the calcium binding protein troponin C, which results in the interaction of the actin–myosin molecules and the generation of force. Relaxation is brought about by the removal of Ca^{2+} from the cytoplasm such that the level drops below the threshold of binding to troponin C and the loss of association between actin and myosin filaments.[1] The cytoplasmic Ca^{2+} concentration is regulated on a beat-to-beat basis by a variety of Ca^{2+} transport systems which are localized in the myocardial cell membrane referred to as the sarcolemma and in the intracellular membrane sarcoplasmic reticulum. A small amount of Ca^{2+} enters the cell via voltage-gated Ca^{2+} channels and, through a positive feedback mechanism, induces substantial Ca^{2+} release from the Ca^{2+} stores of the sarcoplasmic reticulum. The sarcoplasmic reticulum is a specialized tubular network of intracellular membranes that regulates cytoplasmic calcium levels and therefore controls the contraction and relaxation of muscles. The sarcoplasmic reticulum serves a variety of critical functions such as Ca^{2+} release, Ca^{2+} uptake, and Ca^{2+} storage. The structure of the sarcoplasmic reticulum in cardiac muscle is not as well defined as that of the skeletal muscle, especially in relation to the transverse tubules (T-tubules) which are specialized invaginations of the plasma membrane. A simplified cross-sectional view of a cardiac myofiber is shown in Figure 1. The comparatively few transverse tubules in cardiac tissue are of larger diameter and are often coupled on only one side to the terminal cisternae of the sarcoplasmic reticulum to form the dyad junction.[2] Direct coupling of the membranes also occurs between the subcisternae of cardiac sarcoplasmic reticulum and the sarcolemma, which itself constitutes much of the total membrane content of cardiac cells. The sarcoplasmic reticulum membranes contain functionally important proteins such as the Ca^{2+} release channel/ryanodine receptor, Ca^{2+} pump (Ca^{2+}ATPase), and Ca^{2+}-binding protein calsequestrin. These three proteins are characteristic of the sarcoplasmic reticulum and are used as markers to identify and isolate this membrane system. The purified sarcoplasmic reticulum membranes form sealed vesicles of a diameter of 0.1 to 0.2 μm.[3] These vesicles reseal in a right-side-out configuration, most likely because the foot structures/calcium release channels and the complex scaffolding of calsequestrin retain the sarcoplasmic reticulum in a topology which is directly referable to the *in situ* case.

1.1.   Applications

1.1.1. Ca^{2+} transport
Given that purified sarcoplasmic reticulum vesicles contain all of the required machinery in a functional physiological state, they can be used in a wide array

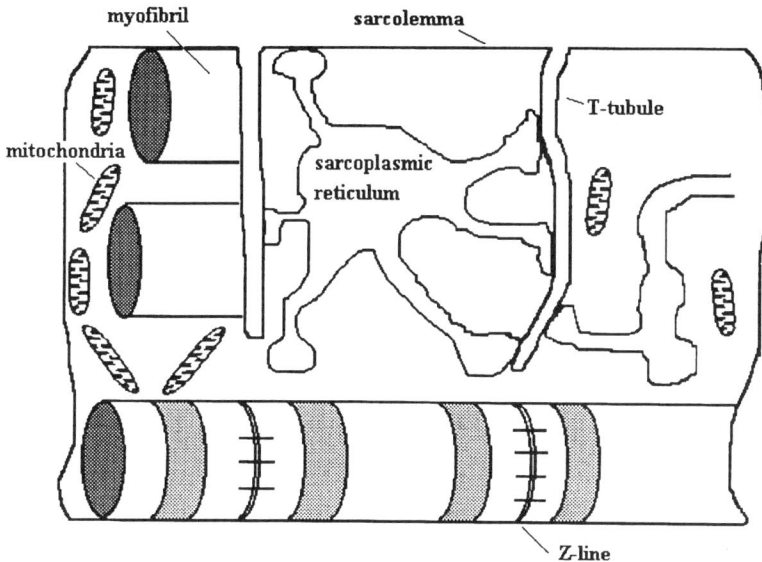

Figure 1
Cross section of a cardiac myofiber.

of investigations on Ca^{2+} transport activities[4,5] (both uptake and release). One application which has proven to be particularly useful is the measurement of oxalate-supported Ca^{2+} accumulation. Using this type of assay, Schwinger et al.[6] have recently provided evidence for reduced Ca^{2+} uptake of sarcoplasmic reticulum from patients with dilated cardiomyopathy, and Labow et al.[7] have studied the effects of hypothermic cardioplegic solutions on energy-mediated Ca^{2+} transport. The method is based on the measurement of radioactive calcium (^{45}Ca) precipitating with oxalate within the sarcoplasmic reticulum vesicles.[4] Following initiation of the reaction, aliquots of the reaction mixture are filtered at various times, and the radioactivity trapped on the filter is determined through liquid scintillation counting. For more detailed information regarding several assays of cardiac Ca^{2+} transport activities, the reader should consult an excellent chapter by Hamilton and Tate.[8]

1.1.2. Protein purification and characterization

The isolation of sarcoplasmic reticulum vesicles provides an excellent starting point for the purification and characterization of its endogenous proteins. Recently cloned proteins, such as the calsequestrin-binding protein junctin,[9] calnexin,[10] and the glucose-regulated protein (GRP94),[11] have been purified and shown to associate with cardiac sarcoplasmic reticulum. Sorcin, a 22-kDa calcium-binding protein, and FKBP12.6, an immunosuppressant binding protein, are two sarcoplasmic reticulum proteins which have been shown to associate specifically with the cardiac ryanodine receptor and may play roles in modulating calcium release channel activity and/or stability.[12,13] The purification and characterization of more novel sarcoplasmic reticulum proteins should continue to provide a better framework for the understanding of sarcoplasmic reticulum function.

1.1.3. Electrophysiology

The activity and gating behavior of the calcium release channel/ryanodine receptor can best be investigated by incorporating purified sarcoplasmic reticulum membranes into lipid bilayers.[14] This is particularly advantageous because the channels retain their native membrane environment which contain a host of regulatory proteins. Hain et al.[15] used this approach to study the effect of exogenous and endogenous kinases on cardiac calcium release channels incorporated into planar lipid membranes.

1.2. Overview of Isolation Procedures

The fractionation procedures employed for the purification of sarcoplasmic reticulum were originally developed for use with skeletal muscle. These same techniques, when applied to cardiac tissue, are not as successful, most probably because of the different structural nature of the cardiac sarcoplasmic reticulum and the predominance of cell surface membranes. The isolation of sarcoplasmic reticulum membranes begins with the homogenization of the heart muscle. The process of homogenization disrupts the sarcolemmal surface and releases the intracellular components from their supporting matrix. Sealed vesicles of the sarcoplasmic reticulum can be purified from the heart muscle homogenate by differential and discontinuous gradient centrifugation. Differential centrifugation separates the released vesicles from the other cellular components (such as nuclei, organelles and cytoskeleton) on the basis of their sedimentation rates. Since the sedimentation rates for sarcolemma and sarcoplasmic reticulum membranes are quite similar, additional procedures such as density gradient centrifugation are often required to separate these two components from each other.

2. Method for Isolating Cardiac Sarcoplasmic Reticulum

The method described below for the isolation of sarcoplasmic reticulum membrane vesicles from pig heart is based on the procedure reported by Meissner and Henderson[5] for canine heart, as modified by Sitsapesan and Williams[16] for sheep heart. To date, the best-characterized sarcoplasmic reticulum preparations have originated from larger animal hearts. Sarcoplasmic reticulum can be obtained from smaller animal hearts and even isolated cardiomyocytes,[17] but usually at the expense of yield or purity. Such adaptations of the purification method have been described for a variety of species including rat,[18] guinea pig,[19] cat,[20] and rabbit.[21]

2.1. Preparation of Solutions

Solution A (2 l)

Add 18 g NaCl (0.9%) and 20 ml of 1 M Tris-HCl, pH 8 (10 mM) to 1.8 l Millipore-purified water.

Adjust the pH of the solution to 8.0.

Add required water for a total volume of 2 l.

Numbers in parentheses indicate final concentrations.

Solution B (1.5 l)

Add 205 g sucrose (0.3 M) and 30 ml of 1 M Pipes, pH 6.8 (20 mM) to 1.3 l Millipore-purified water.

Adjust pH to 7.4.

Add water to a final volume of 1.5 l.

Solution C (500 ml)

Add 15 g KCl (0.4 M), 250 µl of 1 M MgCl$_2$ (0.5 mM), 250 µl of 1 M CaCl$_2$ (0.5 mM), 833 µl of 0.3 M EGTA (0.5 mM), and 10 ml of 1 M Pipes (20 mM), pH 6.8 to 400 ml of Millipore-purified water.

Adjust the pH to 7.0.

Add water to a final volume of 500 ml.

The pH of solutions is measured at room temperature and all solutions are chilled to 4°C prior to use. Protease inhibitors are added to all buffers, just prior to use, in final concentrations of 0.3 mM phenylmethane sulfonyl fluoride (PMSF), 1 mM benzamidine, 1 mM iodoacetamide, and 0.5 µM pepstatin.

2.2. Centrifugation

Two types of centrifugation are employed in the method: differential and discontinuous sucrose density gradient centrifugation. All centrifuges and rotors can be purchased from Beckman Instruments Inc. (Palo Alto, CA). Both rotors and centrifuge chambers are precooled to 4°C prior to centrifugation. The speeds of centrifugation shown are for the specific rotors recommended in this procedure. These can be adjusted for use with any rotor using the following formula:

$$\text{Relative centrifugal force (g)} = 1.12 \text{ r } (\text{rpm}/1000)^2$$

where r is the radius (in mm) of the rotor.

2.2.1. Differential centrifugation of heart homogenates

Differential centrifugation separates particles according to size and density, so that denser particles (i.e. nuclei) will pellet more rapidly than less dense particles (i.e. membrane vesicles). The major difficulty with differential pelleting is that the centrifugal force required to pellet the larger particles from the top of the solution is also sufficient to pellet the smaller particles nearest the bottom of the tube. It is possible to minimize this cross contamination of the pellet by repeated washings. However, this results in loss of the pelleted material. Additionally, some material may be damaged by the repeated resuspension and recentrifugation. Hence, differential pelleting is usually employed for the initial processing of large volumes of homogenates to obtain membrane fractions enriched in the particles of interest prior to further purification. For a more comprehensive coverage of the basic principles of centrifugation, the reader is encouraged to consult a number of excellent sources.[22-24]

Pig hearts obtained from a local abattoir (Abattoir Brisson, Embrun, ON) are transported on ice to the laboratory. If possible, all subsequent procedures are executed in a temperature-controlled cold room (4°C) to minimize proteolytic degradation. Immerse and rinse the heart several times in ice-cold solution A to remove any residual blood within its chambers. There should be no blood present in the final rinse. With a scalpel, trim the ventricular tissue of fat, connective tissue, and surface blood vessels. Chop the tissue with sharp scissors into small (3 cm) cubes. Mince approximately 50-g portions of ventricular tissue in 4 volumes of solution B using 3×5 s pulses of an Osterizer blender (Sunbeam Corp., Canada). If frozen tissue is being used, it can be ground into a fine powder, under liquid nitrogen, using a mortar and pestle and resuspended in the same volume of ice-cold solution B. Homogenize the minced tissue for 3×15 s with a Polytron PT 10/35 homogenizer (Brinkmann Instruments) at half maximal setting, taking care to cool the blades in ice-cold solution B between pulses. Avoid excessive frothing of the homogenate, as some proteins may denature on the surface of the air bubbles. Centrifuge the homogenate for 20 min at 6000 rpm (5500 g max) in a JA-14 rotor. Gently decant the supernatant and filter it through four layers of cheesecloth to remove large unhomogenized particles, insoluble lipids, and denatured proteins. Centrifuge the filtrate for 60 min at 34,000 rpm (135,000 g max) in a Type 35 rotor.

This is a convenient time to prepare the discontinuous sucrose density gradients required for the next purification step. Sucrose is an ideal gradient medium because of its ready availability, stable nature, and inertness towards most biological material.[22] Prepare the three gradient solutions: solution C with either 20, 30, or 40% sucrose (w/v). Remember that these percentages are expressed as weight per volume (w/v); hence the 20% solution will contain 20 g of sucrose in a total volume of 100 ml of solution. When layering the discontinuous density gradients, two approaches can be used. The first involves putting the most dense solution in the bottom of the tube and then overlaying it with next most dense solution. It is somewhat easier and quicker, however, to prepare the gradients, using the underlaying procedure as follows. Using a calibrated syringe fitted with a blunt ended, large-bore needle, carefully introduce 8 ml of the 20% sucrose solution into the bottom of each tube. One discontinuous density gradient should be prepared for each 50 g of starting tissue. Fill a new syringe with 9 ml of 30% sucrose solution. Remove any air bubbles trapped within the syringe. Carefully direct the tip of the needle to the bottom of the tube and underlay the 20% solution with 8 ml of 30% solution. Adjust the delivery of the 30% solution so that interface disturbances are minimized. Repeat the above steps with 8 ml of the 40% sucrose solution. It is useful to indicate the location of the various interfaces with a permanent marker, since these junctions are not always as visible following the centrifugation. Store the discontinuous density gradients at 4°C while you continue with the purification of the heart membranes.

2.2.2. Discontinuous gradient centrifugation of the heart membranes

Discard the supernatant from the 60-min centrifugation step obtained from the differential centrifugation described above. Gently resuspend the pellet in solution C plus 10% sucrose (w/v). Use 4 ml of this solution for each 50 g of starting tissue. Homogenize the pellet using 15 passes of a Potter-Elvehjem tissue grinder with a Teflon pestle (VWR Scientific of Canada Ltd., Toronto, ON). Incubate on ice for 20 min. The potassium chloride in solution C serves to solubilize and remove contaminating actomyosin, stabilize the Ca^{2+} ATPase, and decrease the aggregation of the membranes.[25,26] Centrifuge for 10 min at 6000 rpm (3600 g max) in a 60 Ti rotor to remove large insoluble aggregates. Discard the pellet. Carefully layer 4 ml of supernatant per discontinuous sucrose density gradient using a Pasteur pipette. Verify that opposing tubes are balanced by weighing. Centrifuge gradients for 5 h at 26,000 rpm (122,000 g max) in a SW28 swinging bucket rotor. A swinging bucket rotor is generally recommended when maximum resolution of the sample zones is required. The longer centrifugation times required are offset by the excellent resolution of the sample bands. The rotor should be accelerated slowly, since the greatest potential for disturbing the gradients occurs during the initial acceleration of the rotor from rest. Similarly, swirling of the samples during the deceleration phase of the run can be minimized by letting the rotor coast from 1000 rpm to rest without braking. Many centrifuges offer both of these options as pre-programmed settings. Using a Pasteur pipette, carefully aspirate the sarcoplasmic reticulum membrane vesicles collecting at the 30 to 40% interface and dilute with at least two volumes of solution C. Centrifuge for 45 min at 42,000 rpm (178,000 g max) in a 60 Ti rotor. Discard the supernatant. Gently resuspend the pellets in a total volume of 5 to 10 ml of solution B, using 15 complete passes of a Teflon-glass homogenizer. Save an aliquot (100 µl) for assaying the protein concentration of the sarcoplasmic reticulum vesicles. Rapidly freeze the remaining sample in liquid nitrogen and store at −80°C. The entire purification can be completed on average in about 9 h. A summary of the isolation procedure is shown in Figure 2.

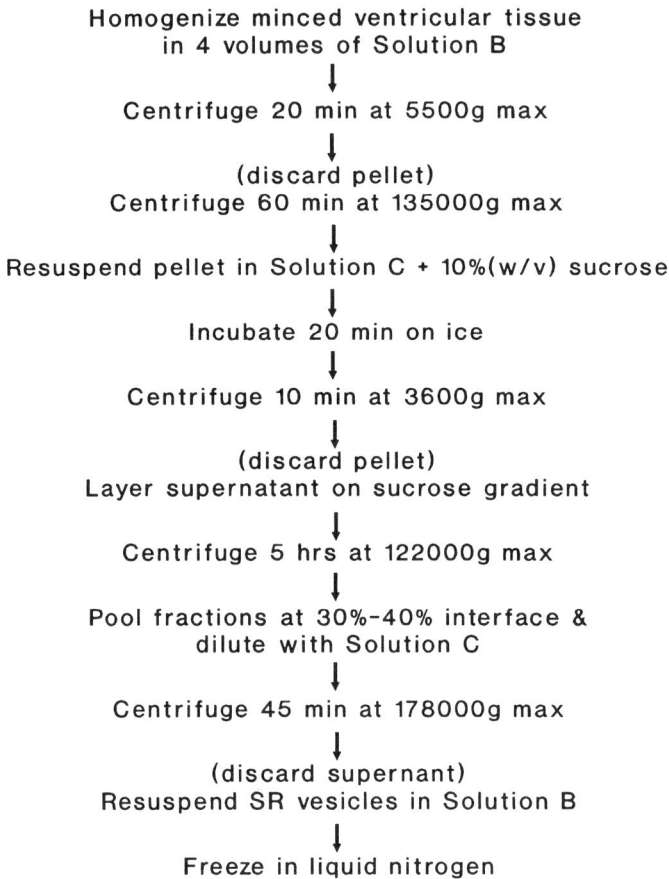

Homogenize minced ventricular tissue
in 4 volumes of Solution B
↓
Centrifuge 20 min at 5500g max
↓
(discard pellet)
Centrifuge 60 min at 135000g max
↓
Resuspend pellet in Solution C + 10%(w/v) sucrose
↓
Incubate 20 min on ice
↓
Centrifuge 10 min at 3600g max
↓
(discard pellet)
Layer supernatant on sucrose gradient
↓
Centrifuge 5 hrs at 122000g max
↓
Pool fractions at 30%–40% interface &
dilute with Solution C
↓
Centrifuge 45 min at 178000g max
↓
(discard supernant)
Resuspend SR vesicles in Solution B
↓
Freeze in liquid nitrogen

Figure 2
Protocol for isolation of cardiac sarcoplasmic reticulum.

2.3. Determination of Purity

2.3.1. [^{3}H] Ryanodine binding assay[27,28]

The identification of the calcium release channel of the sarcoplasmic reticulum is greatly aided by its ability to bind ryanodine, a neutral plant alkaloid.[29] Thus, insight into the purity of a sarcoplasmic reticulum preparation can be gained by following the enrichment of the ryanodine binding sites throughout the purification procedure.

Sarcoplasmic reticulum membranes are washed and resuspended in the following binding solution: 150 mM KCl, 3 mM Na$_2$ATP, 360 μM CaCl$_2$ (60 μM free Ca^{2+}), 10 mM Na-HEPES, pH 7.4, 5 μM PMSF. Protein concentrations are adjusted to approximately 1 mg/ml for the assay. The samples are incubated in triplicate with increasing concentrations (0.1 to 70 nM) of [9,21-^{3}H(N)]-ryanodine (50 to 100 Ci/mmol, DuPont, Mississauga, ON) in a final volume of 1 ml. Nonspecific binding is measured in the presence of a hundredfold excess of unlabeled ryanodine (Calbiochem, La Jolla, CA). The average value of nonspecific binding amounts to 5 to 10% of the total binding of 1 nM [^{3}H] ryanodine.[30] Binding reactions are carried out for 2 h at 37°C. Membrane-bound drug is separated from unbound drug by rapid vacuum filtration through glass fiber filters (Whatman GF/B or Skatron filtermats) using a 12-well cell harvester (Skatron, Sterling, VA). The filters are washed 3 times with 5 ml of binding solution, and radioactivity is measured by liquid scintillation counting. Binding data such as the dissociation constant (K_d) and the maximal binding capacity (B_{max}) can be determined by nonlinear least squares analysis, using programs such as LIGAND.[31]

2.3.2. Other sarcoplasmic reticulum markers

The degree of enrichment of sarcoplasmic reticulum membranes can also be measured through the enrichment of specific marker proteins visible by Coomassie blue staining of the proteins separated by SDS gel electrophoresis. These proteins include the high molecular weight calcium release channel, the predominant Ca^{2+} ATPase, calsequestrin (which stains dark blue with Stains-All) and the 53-kDa glycoprotein.[32]

The degree of contamination of the sarcoplasmic reticulum by sarcolemmal and mitochondrial membranes can be estimated by measuring the activity of specific membrane marker enzymes such as ouabain-sensitive Na$^+$-K$^+$-ATPase[33] and succinate-dehydrogenase,[34] respectively, in the crude homogenate vs. final membrane preparation.

2.4. Examples of Data Obtained

The yield of sarcoplasmic reticulum membranes obtained will vary from animal to animal and depend greatly on the homogenization apparatus used. In our hands, we purify approximately 30 mg of sarcoplasmic reticulum membranes per 100 g of fresh ventricular tissue. The membranes are significantly enriched in sarcoplasmic reticulum vesicles. As shown in Figure 3 (panel A), there is a marked enrichment in sarcoplasmic reticulum (SR) marker proteins such as the ryanodine receptor, Ca^{2+} ATPase, calsequestrin, and 53-kDa glycoprotein as compared to the starting ventricular homogenate (H). Panel B shows an approximate 10-fold enrichment of the ryanodine receptor

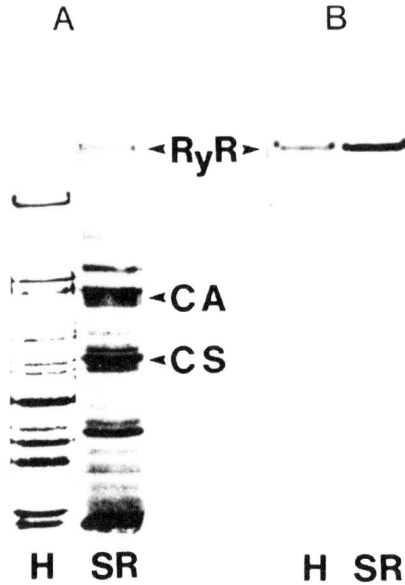

Figure 3

Enrichment of cardiac sarcoplasmic reticulum proteins. Each lane contains 50 μg of porcine heart protein separated by SDS-PAGE and stained with Coomassie brilliant blue R-250 (panel **A**): ventricular homogenate (H); sarcoplasmic reticulum vesicles (SR). The major stained bands corresponding to the ryanodine receptor (RyR), the Ca^{2+}-ATPase (CA), and calsequestrin (CS) are indicated with arrows. The enrichment of the sarcoplasmic reticulum ryanodine receptor was determined by Western blot analysis (panel **B**) of the same cardiac protein samples separated under identical conditions.

as measured by Western-blot analysis using a polyclonal antibody (kindly provided by Dr. D.H. MacLennan) raised against the ryanodine receptor. Equilibrium binding of [^{3}H] ryanodine to the membranes isolated by the aforementioned procedure yielded average values of $B_{max} = 3$ pmol/mg protein and $K_d = 4$ nM for the maximal binding capacity and dissociation constant of the high affinity ryanodine binding site (Figure 4).

2.5.   Potential Problems

Homogenization is perhaps the most crucial step of these preparations, and even slight modifications in the conditions or equipment used can have profound effects on the eventual activity, purity, and yield of the sarcoplasmic reticulum vesicles obtained.[35]

Too long homogenization times, too little homogenization solution, or overheated Polytron blades will result in a homogenate which is gelatinous and fractionates poorly. The homogenization procedure is greatly facilitated

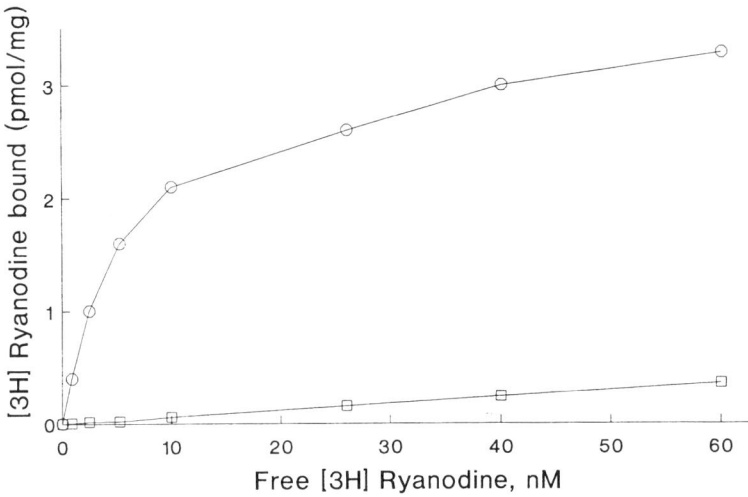

Figure 4

Equilibrium binding of [³H] ryanodine to cardiac sarcoplasmic reticulum membranes. Total binding (○) and nonspecific binding (□) were measured as described in the text. The data were transformed into a Scatchard plot and the dissociation constant (K_d) was 6 nM, and the maximal binding capacity (B_{max}) was 3.2 pmol/mg of protein.

by spending a little extra time to remove most of the fat, connective tissue, valves, blood vessels, and even endocardium from the heart muscle.

This preparation, as well as many variations of the method of Harigaya and Schwartz,[36] can result in sarcoplasmic reticulum vesicles contaminated with up to 15 to 20% sarcolemmal membranes.[37] Several modifications can be made to improve the purity of the sarcoplasmic reticulum membrane preparation isolated above at the expense of the final yield. One method, known as "density augmentation", refers to the selective increase in the density of sarcoplasmic reticulum vesicles brought about by active accumulation of calcium oxalate[38] or calcium phosphate.[39] Separation of the sarcoplasmic reticulum from the contaminating sarcolemma can be achieved, for example, by calcium loading with oxalate which is accumulated via the Ca^{2+} ATPase in the sarcoplasmic reticulum but not in the sarcolemmal vesicles. The drawback of this technique is that it is difficult to remove the loaded calcium oxalate, which can then interfere with the subsequent measurement of calcium transport activities. Alternatively, Chamberlain et al.[33] were successful in employing a linear sucrose density gradient without oxalate loading to enrich sarcoplasmic reticulum vesicles. This procedure, when used with proper attention to details and optimized as described,[35] yields purified cardiac sarcoplasmic reticulum of high quality.

3.   Summary

In summary, this is a relatively versatile and easy method for the isolation of cardiac sarcoplasmic reticulum, which can be applied to a variety of species. There are, of course, many other procedures in the literature which will provide satisfactory isolation of sarcoplasmic reticulum membranes. The method described in this chapter is the one used in our laboratory. It is our hope that this protocol will provide the reader with a simple and efficient method for the preparation of cardiac sarcoplasmic reticulum which can be used in a wide array of cardiovascular research experiments and especially in the study of proteins involved in the regulation of Ca^{2+} uptake and release in cardiomyocytes.

Acknowledgments

This work was supported by a grant from the Heart and Stroke Foundation of Ontario (HSFO). B.S.T. is a career investigator of the HSFO and J.J.L. is the recipient of a Medical Research Council studentship.

References

1. Fozzard, H.A., Excitation-contraction coupling in the heart, *Adv. Exp. Med. Biol.*, 308, 135, 1991.
2. Sommer, J.R. and Jennings, R.B., Ultrastructure of cardiac muscle, in *The Heart and Cardiovascular System: Scientific Foundations*, Fozzard, H. et al., Eds., Raven Press, New York, 1986, 61.
3. DeFoor, P.H., Levitsky, D., Biryukova, T., and Fleischer, S., Immunological dissimilarity of the calcium pump protein of skeletal and cardiac muscle sarcoplasmic reticulum, *Arch. Biochem. Biophys.*, 200, 196, 1980.
4. Sommer, J.R. and Hasselbach, W., The effect of glutaraldehyde and formaldehyde on the calcium pump of the sarcoplasmic reticulum, *J. Cell Biol.*, 34, 902, 1967.
5. Meissner, G. and Henderson, J.S., Rapid calcium release from sarcoplasmic reticulum vesicles is dependent on Ca^{2+} and is modulated by Mg^{2+}, adenine nucleotide and calmodulin, *J. Biol. Chem.*, 262, 3065, 1987.
6. Schwinger, R.H.G., Bohm, M., Schmidt, U., Karczewski, P., Bavendiek, U., Flesch, M., Krause, E.G., and Erdmann, E., Unchanged protein levels of SERCA II and phospholamban but reduced Ca^{2+} uptake and Ca^{2+}-ATPase activity of cardiac sarcoplasmic reticulum from dilated cardiomyopathy patients compared with patients with nonfailing hearts, *Circulation*, 92, 3220, 1995.
7. Labow, R.S., Hendry, P.J., Meek, E., and Keon, W.J., Temperature affects human cardiac sarcoplasmic reticulum energy-mediated calcium transport, *J. Mol. Cell. Cardiol.*, 25, 1161, 1993.

8. Hamilton, S.L. and Tate, C.A., Proteins involved in the uptake and release of Ca²⁺ from the sarcoplasmic reticulum, in *Cellular Calcium*, The Practical Approach Series, McCormack, J.G. and Cobbold, P.H., Eds., Oxford University Press, Toronto, 1991, 313.

9. Jones, L.R., Zhang, L., Sanborn, K., Jorgensen, A.O., and Kelley, J., Purification, primary structure, and immunological characterization of the 26 kDa calsequestrin binding protein (junctin) from cardiac junctional sarcoplasmic reticulum, *J. Biol. Chem.*, 270, 30787, 1995.

10. Cala, S.E., Ulbright, C., Kelley, J.S., and Jones, L.R., Purification of a 90 kDa protein (band VII) from cardiac sarcoplasmic reticulum. Identification as calnexin and localization of casein kinase II phosphorylation sites, *J. Biol. Chem.*, 268, 2969, 1993.

11. Cala, S.E. and Jones, L.R., GRP94 resides within cardiac sarcoplasmic reticulum vesicles and is phosphorylated by casein kinase II, *J. Biol. Chem.*, 269, 5926, 1994.

12. Meyers, M.B., Pickel, V.M., Sheu, S.S., Sharma, V.K., Scotto, K.W., and Fishman, G.I., Association of sorcin with the cardiac ryanodine receptor, *J. Biol. Chem.*, 270, 26411, 1995.

13. Lam, E., Martin, M.M., Timerman, A.P., Sabers, C., Fleischer, S., Lukas, T., Abraham, R.T., O'Keefe, S.J., O'Neill, E.A., and Wiederrecht, G.J., A novel FK506 binding protein can mediate the immunosuppressive effects of FK506 and is associated with the cardiac ryanodine receptor, *J. Biol. Chem.*, 270, 26511, 1995.

14. Sitsapesan, R., Montgomery, R.A., and Williams, A.J., New insights into the gating mechanisms of cardiac ryanodine receptors revealed by rapid changes in ligand concentration, *Circ. Res.*, 77, 765, 1995.

15. Hain, J., Onoue, H., Mayrleitner, M., Fleischer, S., and Schindler, H., Phosphorylation modulates the function of the calcium release channel of sarcoplasmic reticulum from cardiac muscle, *J. Biol. Chem.*, 270, 2074, 1995.

16. Sitsapesan, R. and Williams, A.J., Mechanisms of caffeine activation of single calcium-release channels of sheep cardiac sarcoplasmic reticulum, *J. Physiol.*, 423, 425, 1990.

17. Jones, L.R. and Field, L.J., Residues 2–25 of phospholamban are insufficient to inhibit Ca²⁺ transport ATPase of cardiac sarcoplasmic reticulum, *J. Biol. Chem.*, 268, 11486, 1993.

18. Feher, J.J. and Davis, M.D., Isolation of rat cardiac sarcoplasmic reticulum with improved Ca²⁺ uptake and ryanodine binding, *J. Mol. Cell. Cardiol.*, 23, 249, 1991.

19. Cory, C.R., Grange, R.W., and Houston, M.E., Role of sarcoplasmic reticulum in loss of load-sensitive relaxation in pressure overload cardiac hypertrophy, *Am. J. Physiol.*, 266, H68, 1994.

20. Fujino, S., Satoh, K., Bando, T., Kurokawa, T., Nakai, T., Takashima, K., and Fujino, M., Solubilization and characterization of a ouabain-sensitive protein from transverse tubule membrane-junctional sarcoplasmic reticulum complexes (TTM-JSR) in cat cardiac muscle, *Experientia*, 45, 466, 1989.

21. Hawkins, C., Xu, A., and Narayanan, N., Comparison of the effects of fluoride on the calcium pump of cardiac and fast skeletal muscle sarcoplasmic reticulum: evidence for tissue-specific qualitative difference in calcium-induced pump conformation, *Biochim. Biophys. Acta*, 1191, 231, 1994.

22. *Centrifugation*, 2nd ed., The Practical Approach Series, IRL Press, Washington DC, 1984.

23. Scheeler, P., *Centrifugation in Biology and Medicine*, John Wiley, New York, 1982.

24. de Duve, C., Exploring cells with a centrifuge, *Science*, 189, 186, 1975.

25. Martonosi, A., Sarcoplasmic reticulum. IV. Solubilization of microsomal adenosine triphosphatase, *J. Biol. Chem.*, 243, 71, 1968.

26. MacLennan, D.H., Purification and properties of an adenosine triphosphatase from sarcoplasmic reticulum, *J. Biol. Chem.*, 245, 4508, 1970.

27. Kyselovic, J., Leddy, J.J., Ray, A., Wigle, J., and Tuana, B.S., Temporal differences in the induction of dihydropyridine receptor subunits and ryanodine receptors during skeletal muscle development, *J. Biol. Chem.*, 269, 21770, 1994.

28. Imagawa, T., Smith, J.S., Coronado, R., and Campbell, K.P., Purified ryanodine receptor from skeletal muscle sarcoplasmic reticulum is the calcium permeable pore of the calcium release channel, *J. Biol. Chem.*, 262, 16636, 1987.

29. Lai, F.A., Anderson, K., Rousseau, E., Liu, Q.Y., and Meissner, G., Evidence for a Ca^{2+} channel within the ryanodine receptor complex from cardiac sarcoplasmic reticulum, *Biochem. Biophys. Res. Commun.*, 151, 441, 1988.

30. Pessah, I.N. and Zimanyi, I., Characterization of multiple [^{3}H] ryanodine binding sites on the Ca^{2+} release channel of sarcoplasmic reticulum from skeletal muscle and cardiac muscle: evidence for a sequential mechanism in ryanodine action, *Mol. Pharmacol.*, 39, 679, 1991.

31. Munson, P.J. and Rodbard, D., A versatile computerized approach for characterization of ligand-binding systems, *Anal.Biochem.*, 107, 220, 1980.

32. Lytton, J. and MacLennan, D.H., Sarcoplasmic reticulum, in *The Heart and the Cardiovascular System: Scientific Foundations*, Fozzard, H.A., Ed., Raven Press, New York, 1991, 1203.

33. Chamberlain, B.K., Levitsky, D.O., and Fleischer, S., Isolation and characterization of canine cardiac sarcoplasmic reticulum with improved Ca^{2+} transport properties, *J. Biol. Chem.*, 258, 6602, 1983.

34. Bergmeyer, H.U., *Methods of Enzymatic Analysis*, Weinheim, Deerfield Beach, FL, 1983.

35. Chamberlain, B.K. and Fleischer, S., Isolation of canine cardiac sarcoplasmic reticulum, *Methods Enzymol.*, 157, 91, 1988.

36. Harigaya, S. and Schwartz, A., Rate of calcium binding and uptake in normal animal and failing human cardiac muscle. Membrane vesicles (relaxing system) and mitochondria, *Circ. Res.*, 25, 781, 1969.

37. Jones, L.R., Besch, Jr. H.R., Fleming, J.W., McConnaughey, M.M., and Watanabe, A.M., Separation of vesicles of cardiac sarcolemma from vesicles of cardiac sarcoplasmic reticulum. Comparative biochemical analysis of component activities, *J. Biol. Chem.*, 254, 530, 1979.

38. Jones, L.R. and Cala, S.E., Biochemical evidence for functional heterogeneity of cardiac sarcoplasmic reticulum vesicles, *J. Biol. Chem.*, 256, 11809, 1981.
39. Bonnet, J.P., Galante, M., Brèthes, D., Dedieu, J.C., and Chevallier, J., Purification of sarcoplasmic reticulum vesicles through their loading with calcium phosphate, *Arch. Biochem. Biophys.*, 191, 32, 1978.

Chapter **2**

The Isolation of Myocardial Sarcolemma

Glen F. Tibbits

Contents

1. Introduction 18
    1.1. Uses of Isolated Sarcolemma 18
    1.2. Limitations of the Preparation 19
        1.2.1. SL Recovery 19
        1.2.2. SL Vesicular Size, Orientation, and Integrity 19
    1.3. History of Isolation Procedures 20
2. Methodology 20
    2.1. Starting Material 21
    2.2. Homogenization 21
    2.3. Differential and Sucrose Gradient Centrifugation 22
    2.4. Gradient Fractionation 23
    2.5. Determination of SL Yield, Purification, and Recovery 24
        2.5.1. Assays 24
        2.5.2. Calculations 26
3. Conclusions 27
Acknowledgments 29
References 29

0-8493-3333-4/97/$0.00+$.50
© 1997 by CRC Press, Inc.

17

1. Introduction

Contraction in the mammalian myocardium is regulated by an influx of calcium across the sarcolemma (SL), predominantely through the L-type Ca^{2+} channel, which has been shown to trigger the release of a greater quantity of calcium from the sarcoplasmic reticulum (SR).[1] Despite the fact that the magnitude of Ca^{2+} influx across the SL is less than that released from the SR in the mammalian heart, this transsarcolemmal influx is highly regulated and is one of the main determinants of the magnitude of SR Ca^{2+} release and, therefore, contractility. Furthermore, in the myocardium of lower vertebrates, the SL Ca^{2+} influx may be the only source of contractile calcium.[2] In addition, mechanical relaxation includes SL Ca^{2+} efflux across the sarcolemma primarily through the Na^+-Ca^{2+} exchanger.[3] Thus it is clear that sarcolemma plays a crucial role in the regulation of Ca^{2+} fluxes and, therefore, myocardial contraction and relaxation in all species evaluated. SL Ca^{2+} fluxes, in turn, are regulated in an important way by SL receptors for other ligands, arguably the most important of which is the β adrenergic receptor. In addition, the numerous SL receptors and transporters play critical roles in substrate availability for metabolism and in the response to several growth factors Cardiac sarcolemma plays an important role in the regulation of excitability, contractility, metabolism, and growth and is therefore critical in the regulation of normal cardiac function as well as in the adaptation to both physiological and pathological stressors. As such the sarcolemma has been the focus of numerous investigations. Several different approaches to studying sarcolemmal function can be used, including SL that is largely intact (e.g., whole cell patch clamping) or isolated from the myocyte. Isolated SL can be achieved in several different ways, including: (1) the excised patch,[4] (2) gas dissection,[5] (3) homogenization and affinity purification using conjugated Ab (e.g., Dynall Inc., New Hyde Park, NY) or ligands specific for the SL, and (4) homogenization and differential/sucrose gradient centrifugation. This chapter will focus on the latter, for it is reliable and the equipment required is readily available.

1.1.   Uses of Isolated Sarcolemma

Sarcolemma isolated by differential and sucrose gradient centrifugation in a manner similar in principle to that described in this chapter has been used in a wide variety of studies, a reflection of the numerous functions of the SL. In general these can be divided into three types of investigations, the determination of SL: (1) protein densities, (2) protein characteristics, and (3) lipid composition and membrane physical properties. For each of these studies, the limitations of the preparation as discussed in Section 1.2 must be carefully considered. Once the SL has been isolated and appropriately characterized, it can be the starting point for studies, including but not limited to: ligand binding,[6,7] radioisotopic transport,[8] sodium dodecyl sulfate-polyacrylamide gel electrophoresis (SDS-PAGE),[a] immunoblotting,[9] lipid extraction and thin layer chromatography (TLC) and gas chromatography (GC) on the extracted lipids,[10] lipid extraction and reconstitution of SL proteins into artificial membranes of varying composition.[9,11]

1.2.   Limitations of the Preparation

As with all preparations, one needs to be aware of the limitations in the use of isolated sarcolemma in order that the data can be interpreted correctly. There are two main problems that deserve further discussion: (1) SL recovery, and (2) vesicular size, orientation, and integrity.

1.2.1.   SL recovery

The concept of sarcolemma recovery is absolutely critical when one is comparing the relative amount of a sarcolemmal protein between two different groups. Alterations in the density of SL receptors, transporters, and/or channels are frequently hypothesized as possible mechanisms of cardiac adaptation to a physiological or pathological perturbation. Thus the accurate assessment of protein density is critical in these types of experiments. A major complicating factor in using the isolated SL preparation is that the recovery of the total amount of SL in the SL preparation is relatively low (usually between 5 to 20%) and may be variable. Furthermore, the cross-contamination from other organelles may be relatively high and variable. As a consequence, when the data are normalized per milligram of SL protein, the amount of actual SL protein per milligram of total protein in the preparation may vary. There are two principal ways around this possible caveat. The first is to use crude homogenates to determine densities of SL proteins whenever possible. The crude homogenate preparation represents 100% of the SL as well as other organelles and thus is not affected by differential recoveries. This preparation can be used when: (1) the protein is found only in sarcolemma, and (2) the signal-to-noise ratio is acceptable. Ligand binding to SL receptors can often be performed adequately in crude homogenates. However, for many parameters (e.g., Na^+-Ca^{2+} exchange) the signal-to-noise ratio is not acceptable. The second means of reducing or eliminating the problems with differential recoveries is to carefully assess the SL recovery by using marker enzyme analysis of the fractions recovered from the sucrose gradient. This is discussed in more detail in Section 2.4.1.

1.2.2.   SL vesicular size, orientation, and integrity

When cardiac tissue is disrupted by homogenization, the fragmented organelles tend to form vesicles of varying size, orientation, and integrity. In some types of studies this phenomenon could have a significant bearing on the results. Electron microscopy and other techniques have indicated that the techniques described in this chapter produce SL vesicles with mean diameters of approximately 1 μm. Vesicular size is of importance in two regards. First, in studies in which vesicles are harvested on membranes with fixed pore sizes, it is important that pore size be correct for vesicular size to minimize loss through the filter. Typically we use 0.22 or 0.45 μm for nitrocellulose (e.g., Millipore) membranes and type GF/C for glass-fiber (e.g., Whatman) filters. Second, vesicular size can be important in determining transport rates across SL membranes by affecting intravesicular concentration. The latter is discussed in more detail in Chapter 3 in this book.

After homogenization, the resultant intact vesicles can be classified as inside out (IOV), right side out (ROV), and the remainder being leaky. There are two obvious situations in which vesicular orientation can have a significant impact on the results. The first includes ligand binding studies in which the ligand is lipophobic. In some cases, these problems can be circumvented by osmotically rupturing the vesicles, exposing both sides of the vesicle to the ligand or by changing the ligand to one which is lipophilic. The second situation in which vesicular orientation can be problematic involves the study of transporters which are asymmetric. This problem can be partially addressed by quantifying the percentage of IOV and ROV vesicles by marker enzyme analysis which normally depends on the known asymmetries of the Na^+-K^+ pump.[12] Although there are published techniques to selectively purify vesicles of a specific orientation, none has proven to be reliable. Vesicular integrity can be a serious concern if, for example, determining a transport rate depends on the accumulation of a substrate or end product. The integrity can be evaluated by determining the rate of passive efflux of a substance from the vesicle as we have described.[8] Normally, with the preparation produced from the techniques described in this chapter, the percentage of leaky vesicles is rather low.

1.3. History of Isolation Procedures

The procedures described in this chapter have remained essentially unchanged (with minor improvements) in the last 15 years. Seminal publications by Bers[13] and Reeves and Sutko,[14] both in 1979, brought the SL preparation to a point in which it could yield significant information about sarcolemmal function. Despite this, there are reports published even in recent years with SL preparations that suffer from low purification or unknown purification and recoveries. The dilemma of low purification was circumvented in part by the use of sucrose gradients and the development of the appropriate sucrose densities to physically separate membranes that are SL in origin from those of other organelles.

2. Methodology for Sarcolemmal Isolation

We have used the following procedures to isolate sarcolemma from the hearts of a variety of mammalian (murine,[15] bovine,[16] canine,[9] porcine) and teleost (rainbow trout,[17] skipjack tuna[18]) species. There are subtle variations (e.g., changes in homogenization, layers of the sucrose gradient) that must be used to accommodate species differences. We have also helped to adapt these techniques for the isolation of sarcolemmal from mammalian[19] and fish skeletal muscle with reasonable success. These techniques are based on modifications of that developed by Bers.[13]

2.1. Starting Material

We have used a variety of techniques to sacrifice animals as humanely as possible, all with similar degrees of success. This includes CO_2 poisoning, overdose of sodium pentobarbital, cervical dislocation, and a sharp, rapid blow to the head. In all of the procedures cited above, it is possible and desirable that the heart can still be beating as it is excised. On the other hand, hearts from the slaughterhouse tend not to be good starting material unless one is in a position to receive the heart immediately after the animal has been killed. Also, frozen hearts in general tend not to be good starting material for SL isolation. In addition, one can start the procedure with isolated cardiac myocytes as described in Chapter 7 by Rodrigues and Severson. The advantage of this is that it reduces the contribution of nonmyocyte plasmalemma to the final product. The major disadvantage, of course, is that it makes the isolation procedure much longer and more expensive. Furthermore, because myocytes generally make up about 80% of ventricular wet weight, we have not found contamination of nonmyocyte plasmalemma to be a problem.

For reasonable yields, it is important to start with 5 to 8 g wet weight of heart tissue per isolation. The yield of sarcolemma (in mg SL protein per gram wet weight of heart tissue) decreases outside of this range under the conditions described. Larger starting material masses can be aliquoted into portions of this size, either before or after homogenization. For smaller hearts it is necessary to pool hearts in order to achieve this mass. We have developed a technique to isolate SL from 1.5 to 2 g of heart tissue, but this technique requires a tabletop ultracentrifuge such as the Beckman TLX 100,[19] and although it is technically more demanding, the isolation procedure is also substantially faster.

2.2. Homogenization

After the heart(s) is excised quickly it is then rinsed in a homogenizing medium (HM contains 250 mM sucrose, 20 mM N-tris [hydroxymethyl]-2-2-aminoethanesulfonic acid (TES), pH 7.8 at 21°C) maintained at 4°C. In this medium, the hearts are trimmed of fat, connective tissue, and atria in a shallow well in a blocks of aluminum sitting on ice. We have used several of the Good buffers with equal success including 3-[N-morpholino] propanesulfonic acid (MOPS), HEPES, and TES. One difference between these buffers is the relative sensitivity of the pK_a to temperature. With this factor taken into account, the pH of the solutions described in this chapter can be determined at room temperature (21°C) to yield a pH of ~7.4 at 37°C. The ventricles are then minced with scissors in about 9 to 10 volumes of ice-cold homogenizing medium. The exact value of the final volume is determined in part by the capacity of the tubes for the centrifuge, which in this case equals 51 ml. The myocardia are disrupted further by homogenization using an electric homogenizer. In our lab we use the Tissumizer (Tekmar, Cincinnati, OH), but of course other brands (e.g., Polytron) can be equally effective. The Tissumizer has a built-in timer to control homogenization duration. The degree of homogenization required depends in part on the amount of cardiac connective tissue. In rats, for example, we use setting 40 for 2 bursts of 3 s each. In trout on the other hand, which appears to have little connective tissue, we use setting 30 for one burst of 3 s and setting 20 for another 3-s burst. During the homogenization, it is important to not let the tissue warm because of homogenizer friction. This can be avoided by limiting the duration of homogenization and keeping the tube in an ice bath during the homogenization. The homogenates are then filtered through two layers of wire cloth (nos. 30 and 40 stainless steel) which is available from Small Parts Inc. (Miami Lakes, FL). The filtered homogenate is brought up to the desired final volume with HM. After thorough mixing, a 1 ml aliquot is taken and stored at 4°C for future biochemical analyses, as described in Section 2.2.4.1. Accurate pipetting of this suspension can be tricky as it contains particulate matter which can block the pipette tips. The contractile proteins are rendered soluble by mild KCl (100 mM) and Na$^+$ pyrophosphate (25 mM) treatment.

Note: *We keep a stock solution of 1 M KCl and 250 mM Na$^+$ pyrophosphate.*

Thus, to the remaining 50 ml of homogenate, we add 5.5 ml of this KCl/Na$^+$ pyrophosphate solution. This suspension can either be covered with Parafilm and inverted several times or stirred at 4°C for several minutes. This suspension is separated into two aliquots of ~28 ml each in thick-walled polycarbonate ultracentrifuge tubes.

2.3.   Differential and Sucrose Gradient Centrifugation

The tubes are spun at 180,000 × g (we use the Beckman Ti 50.2 rotor) on an ultracentrifuge for 1 h at 4°C. The supernatants from this spin, which should contain the cytosolic proteins as well as the solubulized contractile proteins, are discarded. The pellets are resuspended in 20 ml of ice-cold HM by gently using a motor-driven Teflon pestle followed by a one-time 3 s burst at setting 20 of the Tissumizer. For myocardia from species with less connective tissue (e.g., trout), this last step with the Tissumizer is omitted. The resultant suspension is then spun at 2000 × g for 15 min (we use the Beckman J21C rotor) to pellet heavier cellular components. Unfortunately, sometimes SL may be attached to some of the heavier components (e.g., stands of DNA), resulting in loss of SL at this or a later step. In this case, treatment with DNase prior to the low speed spin (as originally proposed by Philipson et al. and modified for our needs[15]) can significantly improve yield and recovery. The supernatants are carefully removed and placed into tubes for the ultracentrifuge and the pellets are discarded. The supernatants are spun at $180,000 \times g$ for 1 h in the ultracentrifuge. The resultant pellet is resuspended in 5 ml of 45% (541 g/l) sucrose, using a Teflon pestle, and the viscous suspension is placed on the bottom of a thick-walled polycarbonate tube for the swing bucket rotor (e.g., Beckman SW28) to be used. A discontinuous sucrose gradient is then made on top of the 45% sucrose by sequentially layering 5 ml each of 32, 30, and 28% sucrose steps.

Note: *We have tried using the polymers (e.g., Ficoll, Percoll) that are commercially available, which allow one to establish the appropriate gradient of densities while minimizing the osmotic gradient. It should be noted that even a 28% sucrose solution is several fold greater than the "normal" tonicity of physiological solutions of ~300 mOsM. However, there are no obvious benefits in our hands in terms of sarcolemmal function, and the isolation becomes substantially more expensive.*

The layering is done while the tube is on ice using a Pasteur pipette and gently adding the sucrose down the side of the tube about 5 mm above the surface to prevent turbulence and mixing of the layers. This can be practiced by artificially coloring the sucrose of different concentrations in order that the steps can be more readily visualized. We keep 5-ml aliquots of each sucrose concentration at $-20°C$. A layer of 8% sucrose is added on top of the 28% sucrose with sufficient volume to bring the gradient to the appropriate volume for centrifugation as dictated by the tube type and the manufacturer. The gradients are then spun in a swing bucket rotor at $122,000 \times g$ overnight (~16 h) in the ultracentrifuge. Although it may not be crucial, we accelerate and decelerate the gradients slowly in the centrifuge.

2.4. Gradient Fractionation

After carefully removing the tubes from buckets, observe the gradients against a dark backdrop. Typically, one should see a whitish band near the 8/28% interface, another band of white-yellow coloration about 5 to 10 mm below this, and a third that has a distinct brownish hue at or near the bottom of the tube. The bands in the tube can be marked with a felt pen for clarity when fractionating the gradient. The first fraction (F1) includes sucrose solution from the top of the tube to just above the first band and is carefully removed with a Pasteur pipette, ensuring that the bands are not disturbed. The second fraction (F2) will include all of the remaining solution above the first band and enough of the solution below to ensure that all of this band is removed without disturbing the band below. F2 is the sarcolemmal fraction, and this fact should be reflected in the marker enzyme analyses done later. In all, the gradient is fractionated into four tubes, labeled F1 to F4 in order of increasing densities. All fractions are maintained at 4°C and diluted with roughly equal volumes of an ice-cold solution of 560 mM NaCl and 40 mM TES (4× LM — see below) in order to avoid osmotic shock. The tubes are allowed to equilibrate for approximately 30 to 60 min on ice, after which they are slowly diluted with an ice-cold loading medium (LM) which contains 140 mM NaCl and 10 mM TES (pH 7.8 at 21°C). The Na$^+$ used in this loading solution is used to facilitate Na$^+$-Ca^{2+} exchange determinations done at a later date, but the loading solution can be changed in order to accommodate other experiments. The diluted fractions are then centrifuged at 180,000 × g for 1 h at 4°C (Ti50.2 rotor), in order to pellet the membranes. In our experience, F1 contains virtually no protein, and thus we routinely discard it prior to this centrifugation step; however, it is worth checking several times in the beginning. The pellets from F2 and F3 are then resuspended in 1.0 to 1.5 ml LM to give a final protein concentration of 1.5 to 4 mg · ml. F4, which has a much higher protein content, can be resuspended in greater volumes of LM. All fractions are characterized as described below and then frozen in liquid N$_2$. While the freezing and storing of highly purified sarcolemma at –195°C for periods of least 6 months has no effect on any sarcolemmal function that we routinely measure (e.g., Na$^+$-Ca^{2+} exchange; K$^+$ pNPPase — see below), this should be checked for other assays that you will perform.

2.5. Determination of SL Yield, Purification, and Recovery

The homogenate which has been stored overnight in the refrigerator can now be compared to the fractions that are harvested from the gradient. We find that after 10 to 24 h at 4°C, the homogenate shows no loss of protein or K$^+$-stimulated p-nitrophenylphosphatase (K$^+$$p$NPPase) activity. It is more efficient to run all of the assays simultaneously on the 2nd day, and so this procedure is strongly recommended.

2.5.1. Assays
For protein determinations on all fractions, we use the method of Bradford,[20] using 20 μg of BSA as a standard (Table 1). Of course, one should construct a standard curve which in our hands is linear from <1 μg to ~40 μg protein. A kit can be purchased from Bio-Rad; however we make our own solutions, which are simple, stable for at least 2 weeks, and substantially less expensive than the kit. One potential drawback to this assay is the very high (~0.550) blank OD. Other assays (e.g., modified Lowry, Biuret) can probably serve equally well. We use the sarcolemmal marker K$^+$$p$NPPase in order to determine SL yield, purification, and recovery (Table 2). This enzyme is a component

TABLE 1
Protein Assay Recipe

	Aliquots (in μl) added to each tube					
	Blank	STD	HMG	F2	F3	F4
DDW[a]	100	90	90	90	90	90
BSA[b] Std	—	10	—	—	—	—
Samples	—	—	10*	10	10	10*
Bradford dye	5,000	5,000	5,000	5,000	5,000	5,000
Total	5,100	5,100	5,100	5,100	5,100	5,100

Stock Solutions

BSA   2 mg/ml (kept at 4°C and monitored by OD of standard which should be ~0.250)

Bradford dye   Made according to Bradford and kept at room temperature in a dispenser bottle for 2–4 weeks.

Samples   *Note the 1:10 dilutions as specified in the worksheet

Steps

1. It is important to add the 90 μl of DDW to the test tubes first
2. Both the BSA standard and the samples should be added directly to the 90 μl aliquot of DDW in the bottom of the tube and not allowed to run down the sides of the tube
3. After the Bradford dye is added, each tube is vortexed and then allowed to stand at room temperature for 5–10 min for color development
4. The tubes are read at 595 nm

[a] DDW, double-distilled water or its equivalent.

[b] BSA, bovine serum albumin.

of the Na^+-K^+ ATPase but is simpler to measure and in general yields more consistent results. We run both of these assays in 13×100-mm disposable test tubes which fit directly in our spectrophotometric sample well for expediency and with reasonable consistency in the triplicates. However, standard spectroscopic-grade cuvettes may also be used. We have adapted both of these assays as well as others for SL characterization for use with a microplate reader.[19] The major advantage is the substantial (4 to 8×) reduction in the amount of sarcolemmal protein used to characterize the preparation. The development process was largely a proportional scaling down of the assay volumes as described in this chapter. The disadvantage is that it requires considerably more diligence and expertise to achieve consistent and reproducible results.

The $K^+pNPPase$ assay as shown in Table 2 is set up to determine the K^+-dependent component of the $pNPPase$ activity by using ±100 mM (final concentration) KCl. Perhaps a preferable determination would be to include 100 μM ouabain in the –K^+ column. The reason that we do not normally do this is that we use these isolation procedures most frequently in the rat heart, which is insensitive to ouabain. However, in preparations which are not anomalous in this regard, the results are essentially the same, regardless whether one uses –K^+ or +ouabain. Furthermore, it should be pointed out that

TABLE 2
K+pNPPase Assay Recipe

	Blank	STD	+K	–K
Aliquots (in µl) added to each tube				
DDW	600	550	580	580
p-Nitrophenol	—	50	—	—
Rx medium	200	200	200	200
KCl	—	—	100	—
NaCl	100	100	—	100
Samples	—	—	20*	20*
pNPPO$_4$	100	100	100	100
Total	1,000	1,000	1,000	1,000

Stock solutions

p-Nitrophenol	50 µM (K+pNPPase reaction end product) is kept at –20°C)
Rx medium	5 mM MgCl$_2$; 1 mM EGTA[a]; 50 mM [MOPS or TES] to give pH 7.0 at 37°C
KCl	500 mM
NaCl	500 mM
pNPPO$_4$	50 mM (K+pNPPase reaction substrate) is kept at –20°C in appropriate aliquot sizes)
Samples	*Note the 1:10 dilution factors from the worksheet

Steps
1. Keep tubes on ice during pipetting
2. Add DDW first and substrate (pNPPO$_4$) last
3. Incubate at 37°C for 20 min
4. Take out and put rack immediately in an ice water slurry to slow reaction
5. Add 2 ml 1 N NaOH to each tube to stop reaction and facilitate color development
6. Remove from ice and allow tubes to reach room temperature
7. Wipe tubes dry and read OD at 415 nm

[a] EGTA, ethyleneglycol-bis-(B-aminoethyl ether)-N,N,N′,N′-te-traacetic acid.

we have used essentially only these two assays for many years with some confidence. However, this is only after having first characterized the preparation more exhaustively with a battery of marker enzymes for SL as well as other organelles.

2.5.2. Calculations

We use a Microsoft Excel spreadsheet for all of the calculations that are derived from these assays. Once the template is set up and the data are entered, all the calculations are performed automatically and the results can be displayed clearly and consistently for each sample. An example of the spreadsheet output using rat heart as starting material is shown in Figure 1. From the display of this worksheet and a description of the calculations to be made (as described), it should be relatively straightforward to construct a worksheet tailored to your applications.

Notes: *However, if you do not have this capability, the templates can be sent to you. Send a blank PC-formatted 3.5″ floppy disk and SASE to: Cardiac Membrane Research Laboratory, Simon Fraser University, Burnaby, BC, V5A 1S6, Canada.*

From the Bradford Assay

1. From the homogenate, fraction, and BSA standard ODs, calculate homogenate and fraction [protein].

2. From the homogenate and fraction [protein] and the total volume of each calculate the total protein content of the homogenate and fractions.

3. Express the total homogenate and fraction protein content per gram wet weight of starting material. This value for the homogenate should be ~10% or 100 ± 15 mg protein per gram wet wt in the mammalian heart. This value for the fractions gives the yield. As F2 should be the sarcolemmal fraction, this value for F2 will be the SL yield, and typically should be in the range of 0.3 to 1.5 mg protein per gram wet wt.

From the K⁺pNPPase Assay

4. From the homogenate, fractions, and standard ODs, calculate the amount (in nmol) of end product produced in each tube.

5. From these values calculate the amount produced per milligram protein and per hour incubation for each tube. These values represent the specific K⁺pNPPase activity. For the homogenate, typically these are in the range of 0.2 to 0.7 µmol/mg protein per hour.

6. For each fraction, calculate the purification index (PI), which is the ratio of the specific K⁺pNPPase activity in each fraction over that in the homogenate. The PI in F2 should be the highest of all fractions and in the range of 10 to 40. If this is not the case, it suggests the gradient was not fractionated correctly.

7. For each fraction and the homogenate, determine the product of the specific K⁺pNPPase activity and total protein.

8. To determine sarcolemmal recovery (R), express this product (described in step 7) for the fractions as a percentage of that in the homogenate. For F2, this value should be in the range of 8 to 20%.

3. Conclusions

The method for sarcolemmal isolation described in this chapter uses differential and sucrose gradient centrifugation. The preparation can be used for a variety of analyses of sarcolemmal function in the heart, including the

PROTEIN ASSAY EXP ID R2305 DATE 25-Jan-96

	HMG	amount		
HMG		56.0 ml	EXP ID	R2305
F1	F1	1.5 ml	wet wt	6.04 g
F2	F2	1.5 ml	Blank OD	0.541
F3	F3	1.5 ml		
F4	F4	2.0 ml		

	dilution factor	aliquot vol µl	OD	OD	OD	mean	µg	mg/ml	mg	yield mg/g
STD			0.250	0.265	0.260	0.258	20.00			
HMG	10	10	0.136	0.130	0.132	0.133	10.27	10.27	575.17	95.23
F1	1	10	0.020	0.005	0.010	0.012	0.90	0.09	0.14	0.02
F2	1	10	0.334	0.323	0.319	0.325	25.19	2.52	3.78	0.63
F3	1	10	0.450	0.465	0.452	0.456	35.28	3.53	5.29	0.88
F4	10	10	0.240	0.248	0.265	0.251	19.43	19.43	38.86	6.43

K^+ pNPPase ASSAY incub 20 min temp 37°C

	dilution factor	aliquot vol µl	µg	OD	OD	mean	nmol	nmol/hr	µmol/ mg/hr	µmol/h	PI	R
STD		50		0.270	0.262	0.265	50.0					
HMG +K	10	20	20.54	0.042	0.040	0.041						
HMG −K				0.020	0.022	0.021						
HMG ΔK						0.020	3.72	11.15	0.54	312.09	1.0	100.0
F2 +K	10	20	5.04	0.155	0.152	0.156						
F2 −K				0.055	0.049	0.051						
F2 ΔK						0.104	19.71	59.13	11.74	44.35	21.6	14.2
F3 +K	1	20	70.55	0.546	0.557	0.552						
F3 −K				0.115	0.112	0.000						
F3 ΔK						0.552	104.28	312.85	4.43	23.46	8.2	7.5
F4 +K	10	20	38.86	0.070	0.071	0.070						
F4 −K				0.020	0.021	0.021						
F4 ΔK						0.049	9.32	27.96	0.72	27.96	1.3	9.0

Figure 1
SL isolation worksheet.

characterization of membrane transport, receptor ligand interactions, and membrane physical properties. However, concern must be paid to the limitations that this preparation imposes, and these are discussed in some detail. Assays used in the characterization of sarcolemmal cross contamination, yield, recovery, and purification are described. The specific use of this preparation in the analysis of Na^+-Ca^{2+} exchange is described in Chapter 3.

Acknowledgments

The comments and suggestions of Dr. Louise Milligan concerning this chapter are appreciated. The author gratefully acknowledges grant support from the Heart and Stroke Foundation of British Columbia and Yukon and NSERC of Canada.

References

1. Fabiato, A., Calcium-induced release of calcium from the cardiac sarcoplasmic reticulum, *Am. J. Physiol.,* 245, C1–C14, 1983.
2. Tibbits, G.F., Hove-Madsen, L., and Bers, D.M., Ca^{2+} transport and the regulation of cardiac contractility in lower vertebrates, *Can. J. Zool.,* 69, 2014–2019, 1991.
3. Bers, D.M. and Bridge, J.H.B., Relaxation of rabbit ventricular muscle by Na-Ca exchange and sarcoplasmic reticulum calcium pump, *Circ. Res.,* 65, 334–342, 1989.
4. McLarnon, J.G., Hamman, B.N., and Tibbits, G.F., Temperature dependence of unitary properties of an ATP-dependent potassium channel in cardiac myocytes, *Biophys. J.,* 65, 2013–2020, 1993.
5. Post, J.A., Langer, G.A., Op den Kamp, J.A.F., and Verkleij, A.J., Phospholipid assymetry in cardiac sarcolemma. Analysis of intact cells and "gas dissected" membranes, *Biochim. Biophys. Acta,* 943, 256–266, 1988.
6. Glossmann, H., Ferry, D.R., Goll, A., and Rombusch, M., Molecular pharmacology of the calcium channel: evidence for subtypes, multiple drug-receptor sites, channel subunits, and the development of a radioiodinated 1,4-dihydropyridine calcium channel label, [^{125}I]iodipine, *J. Cardiovasc. Pharmacol.,* 6, S608–S6121, 1984.
7. Colvin, R.A., Ashavaid, T.F., and Herbette, L.G., Structure-function studies of canine cardiac sarcolemmal membranes. I. Estimation of receptor site densities, *Biochim. Biophys. Acta,* 812, 601–608, 1985.
8. Tibbits, G.F. and Philipson, K.D., Na+-dependent alkaline earth metal uptake in cardiac sarcolemmal vesicles, *Biochim Biophys. Acta,* 817, 327–332, 1985.
9. Tibbits, G.F., Philipson, K.D., and Kashihara, H., Characterization of myocardial Na^+-Ca^{2+} exchange in rainbow trout, *Am. J. Physiol.,* 262, C411–C417, 1992.
10. Tibbits, G.F., Sasaki, M., Nagatomo, T., and Barnard, R.J., Cardiac sarcolemma: compositional adaptation to exercise, *Science,* 213, 1271–1273, 1981.

11. Vemuri, R. and Philipson, K.D., Phospholipid composition modulates the Na+-Ca2+ exchange activity of cardiac sarcolemma in reconstituted vesicles, *Biochim. Biophys. Acta,* 937, 258–268, 1988.

12. Caroni, P. and Carafoli, E., The regulation of the Na+-Ca2+ exchanger of heart sarcolemma, *Eur. J. Biochem.,* 132, 451–460, 1983.

13. Bers, D.M., Cardiac sarcolemma: isolation and characterization, *Biochim. Biophys. Acta,* 555, 131–146, 1979.

14. Reeves, J.P. and Sutko, J.L., Sodium-calcium exchange in cardiac sarcolemmal vesicles, *Proc. Natl. Acad. Sci. U.S.A.,* 76, 590–594, 1979.

15. Tibbits, G.F., Sasaki, M., Ikeda, M., Shimada, K., Tsuruhara, T., and Nagatomo, T., Characterization of rat myocardial sarcolemma, *J. Mol. Cell. Cardiol.,* 13, 1051–1061, 1981.

16. Shi, Z.Q., Davison, A.J., and Tibbits, G.F., Effects of active oxygen generated by DTT/Fe2+ on cardiac Na+/Ca2+ exchange and membrane permeability to Ca2+, *J. Mol. Cell. Cardiol.,* 21, 1009–1016, 1989.

17. Tibbits, G.F., Kashihara, H., Thomas, M.J., Keen, J.E., and Farrell, A.P., Ca2+ transport in myocardial sarcolemma from rainbow trout, *Am. J. Physiol.,* 259, R453–R460, 1990.

18. Tibbits, G.F., Kashihara, H., and Brill, R.W., Myocardial sarcolemma isolated from skipjack tuna, *Katsuwonus pelamis, Can. J. Zool.,* 70, 1240–1245, 1992.

19. Tibbits, G.F., Milligan, L., and Little, S., Rapid isolation of sarcolemma from small hearts, in preparation.

20. Bradford, M., A rapid and sensitive method for the quantitation of microgram quantities of protein utilizing the principle of protein-dye binding, *Anal. Biochem.,* 72, 248–254, 1976.

Chapter **3**

Measurement of Na$^+$-Ca^{2+} Exchange

Glen F. Tibbits

Contents

1. Introduction 32
    1.1. Methods of Measurement of Cardiac Na$^+$-Ca^{2+} Exchange 32
    1.2. Limitations of the Measurement 33
        1.2.1. SL Vesicles 33
        1.2.2. *In Vitro* Measurement 34
    1.3. History of Na$^+$-Ca^{2+} Exchange Procedures 34
2. Measurement of Na$^+$-Ca^{2+} Exchange in Cardiac SL Vesicles 34
    2.1. Starting Material 34
    2.2. Na$^+$-Dependent Ca^{2+} Uptake 35
    2.3. Time Dependence 38
    2.4. Ca^{2+} Concentration Dependence 38
    2.5. Passive Efflux 39
    2.6. Calculations 40
        2.6.1. Worksheet 40
3. Conclusions 42
Acknowledgments 42
References 42

1.   Introduction

Na$^+$-Ca^{2+} exchanger proteins are found in the plasma membranes of many tissues.[5,13,18] In cardiac muscle, this exchanger is a sarcolemmal protein which plays an important role in the regulation of cytosolic [Ca^{2+}] and, therefore, of myocardial contractility.[13,14,18] Since the cloning of the cardiac Na$^+$-Ca^{2+} exchanger in 1990 by Philipson and co-workers,[11] much has been learned about the molecular structure of this protein in relation to its function. In the mammalian heart, the process of excitation-contraction coupling is mediated by a transsarcolemmal influx of Ca^{2+} to trigger the release of Ca^{2+} from the sarcoplasmic reticulum.[6] The best documented role for the exchanger is the beat-to-beat removal of Ca^{2+} from the cytosol to the interstitial space. Although it is known that there are two proteins that could potentially play this role, the Na$^+$-Ca^{2+} exchanger and the SL Ca^{2+} pump, in physiological experiments it is difficult to document a substantive role for the pump. In corroboration, it has been shown that the Na$^+$-Ca^{2+} exchanger is important in the mechanical relaxation of the mammalian heart.[1,4] Both in the hearts of primitive species such as the amphibians and teleosts and during early ontogeny of some mammalian species, it appears that all of the contractile Ca^{2+} comes across the sarcolemma, and relaxation involves purely a transsarcolemmal efflux of Ca.$^{2+}$ In studies from these species, the role of the exchanger is paramount. In addition to the well-documented role of the exchanger in the efflux of Ca,$^{2+}$ there have also been suggestions that the exchanger also contributes to the influx of Ca^{2+} and plays a role in Ca^{2+}-induced Ca^{2+} release.[9]

1.1.   Methods of Measurement of Cardiac Na$^+$-Ca^{2+} Exchange

There have been several different means of measuring Na$^+$-Ca^{2+} exchange in cardiac muscle. These techniques can be divided into measurements of two types: (1) radioisotopic fluxes of Ca^{2+} and/or Na$^+$ or (2) ionic currents using electrophysiological techniques. Radioisotopic flux studies were first done on intact cells, and this approach provided the first evidence of the cardiac Na$^+$-Ca^{2+} exchanger in 1968.[20] With the advent of procedures to isolate relatively pure sarcolemma, this preparation has been the one of choice for the radio-isotopic method, because of the control over conditions that it affords the investigator. This is the procedure that is described in some detail in this chapter. Similarly, the electrophysiological approach has been used on intact tissue, isolated myocytes, and isolated sarcolemma through the giant excised patch procedure. The problems with the electrophysiological techniques have included (1) lack of voltage control (not spaced clamped), (2) currents of mixed origin that were difficult to dissect without a specific blocker of the Na$^+$-Ca^{2+} exchanger, and (3) lack of access to T-tubular spaces. Many of these problems have been resolved using the giant excised patch as developed by Hilgemann,[7] and thus this technique has yielded considerable information about the regulation of the exchanger. However, this technique is extremely demanding technically and can only be performed in a handful of laboratories. Its sophistication precludes it from becoming a routine measurement to most investigators interested in pursuing hypotheses that involve potential adaptation of the Na$^+$-Ca^{2+} exchanger. As such, this chapter focuses on the measurement of cardiac sodium–calcium exchanger activity using the radioisotopic method on isolated sarcolemmal vesicles.

1.2. Limitations of the Measurement

As with all preparations, one needs to be aware of the limitations in the use of isolated sarcolemma to determine Na$^+$-Ca^{2+} exchange activity. The major problems in using isolated SL are of two types: those that are related to the vesicular nature of isolated SL and those related to the fact that this is an *in vitro* measurement in which possible regulatory influences may have been disrupted by the isolation procedure.

1.2.1. SL vesicles

The main issues in the vesicular nature of isolated sarcolemma that can have a bearing on the measurement of Na$^+$-Ca^{2+} exchange are: vesicular leakiness, volume, and orientation. Leakiness has an effect on the ability for the vesicles to retain Ca^{2+}, and vesicular Ca^{2+} content is the basis of this measurement. The small vesicular volumes (0.1 to 0.5 μm diameters) can result in high intravesicular concentrations being achieved in relatively short periods of time precluding one from observing initial rates. This may be addressed adequately by quenching the reaction, as described below, at early times (0.5 to 3 s). However, if the vesicular volumes are extremely small, one may have to resort to other techniques including using proteoliposomes with EGTA[8] included to minimize increases in [Ca^{2+}]$_i$ in order to measure true initial rates.

The third problem is associated with vesicular orientation. Although sarcolemmal isolation procedures result in vesicles that are both right side (ROV) and inside (IOV) out, the technique that is described in this chapter apparently measures only the Na$^+$-Ca^{2+} exchange activity of the IOV population.[10] This conclusion is based on studies which demonstrate an asymmetry of the Ca^{2+} binding sites on the two sites of the membrane, with the high and low affinity sites being on the cytosolic and extracellular sides, respectively. Thus, over the range of extravesicular Ca^{2+} concentrations used in these procedures (5 to 200 μM), only the high affinity site is occupied by Ca^{2+}, so that in the comparison of cardiac Na$^+$-Ca^{2+} exchange activities between two groups, differential vesicular orientation could be a factor in the interpretation of the results.

1.2.2.   In vitro measurement

The isolated sarcolemma preparation, while convenient for measurement of Na^+-Ca^{2+} exchange, may lack regulatory influences that may be important as determined by other methods of measurement. For example, experiments using voltage clamp on the giant excised patch preparation indicate regulation of the exchanger by both Ca^{2+} and ATP,[7] neither of which is observed in isolated vesicles. Also the K_m (Ca^{2+}), although easiest to measure in SL vesicles, often exhibits higher values (10 to 50 μM), which reflect lower affinities, in the SL preparation than that observed with other preparations.

1.3.   History of Na^+-Ca^{2+} Exchange Procedures

Na^+-Ca^{2+} exchange was first determined in cardiac muscle by Reuter and Seitz in 1968,[20] using radioisotopic fluxes in guinea pig atria. It was first measured in cardiac sarcolemmal vesicles by Reeves and Sutko in 1979,[19] and the procedures that are described in this chapter have their bases in that original publication. This technique, which is relatively straightforward, is normally the method of choice because of its simplicity. However, the limitations that are described above must be carefully considered. Since 1979, a tremendous amount of information about the cardiac Na^+-Ca^{2+} exchanger has been collected, using similar procedures to determine: stoichiometry,[17] substrate specificity,[22] and the effects of proteases,[15] free radical-generating systems,[16,21] temperature,[3,23] membrane lipid composition,[24] ischemia,[2] and pH[12] on the exchanger. Thus this approach has proven to be invaluable in our understanding of the role of this protein in cardiac function and will continue to be, as long as the limitations of this procedure are kept in mind in designing experiments.

2.   Measurement of Na^+-Ca^{2+} Exchange in Cardiac SL Vesicles

2.1.   Starting Material

Normally the starting material for these experiments is highly purified cardiac sarcolemmal vesicles that are preloaded with 140 mM NaCl (Table 2a). The preparation of vesicles for these measurements is described in Chapter 2 of this volume. The main criteria are to have sufficiently high $^{45}Ca^{2+}$ content after the exchange reaction to be measurable and for this to be significantly higher than that of the blank. In other words, the signal-to-noise ratio must be acceptable. This precludes, in general, the use of crude SL preparations. As starting material, one may also use reconstituted vesicles in which the native lipid bilayer has been replaced with asolectin or membranes of controlled phospholipid composition. Studies of this type have been extremely important in the investigation of the effect of lipid bilayer constituents on exchanger function, and it should be noted that the effect is robust. Also, this technique has been used to determine if differences in exchanger function between two groups are due to changes in bilayer composition or the protein itself.

For native vesicles of reasonable purification, typically the protein concentration should be in the range of 1.5 to 4 mg/ml. If the protein concentration is too low, (1) the bead of SL that is placed on the wall of the polystyrene tube may not adhere well enough to control initiation of the reaction, and (2) the signal-to-noise ratio may be too low. Protein concentrations which are too high are a waste of starting material and may also influence the $[Ca^{2+}]_o$ in the tube by an intravesicular sequestration which is too large. The percent uptake of total extravesicular Ca^{2+} into the vesicle can be calculated of course, and perhaps this parameter could be included as a column in the worksheet.

2.2.   Na$^+$-Dependent Ca^{2+} Uptake

Na$^+$-Ca^{2+} exchange in this procedure is measured as the sodium-dependent calcium uptake into the vesicles as a function of time or $[Ca^{2+}]_o$. To control the initiation of the reaction, normally a 5-μl drop of SL is placed on the wall of a 3.5 ml (12 × 55 mm) polystyrene tube about 5 mm above the 245 μl of reaction medium. The constituents of the reaction media are shown in Table 1. For all data points, there are two different reaction media that contain 140 mM of either KCl or NaCl (Table 1a). The Ca^{2+} uptake in the Na$^+$-loaded SL vesicles that are diluted into 140 mM KCl is largely that of Na$^+$-Ca^{2+} exchange, as in this condition a large outwardly directed Na$^+$ concentration gradient is rapidly established. In contrast, there is no Na$^+$ gradient in vesicles diluted into 140 mM NaCl. Thus the uptake by vesicles diluted into NaCl represents blanks, and the counts should be subtracted for all data points. This allows for the correction of ^{45}Ca^{2+} that is bound superficially to the sarcolemma or permeates the vesicle by some pathway other than Na$^+$-Ca^{2+} exchange. In general, this Ca^{2+} uptake should be no greater than 10% of that obtained with K$^+$ dilution.

Valinomycin, a K$^+$ ionophore, is used to establish an inside positive transvesicular membrane potential in the SL vesicles that are diluted into 140 mM KCl because of the large inward directed K$^+$ concentration gradient. As the stoichiometry of the Na$^+$-Ca^{2+} exchanger is 3 Na$^+$ per Ca,$^{2+}$ the exchanger is electrogenic and as such is sensitive to membrane potential. The exchanger activity in these vesicles results in an outward current and the inside positive potentials stimulate the exchanger activity.

The reaction is initiated by the addition of SL to the reaction media and is terminated after a fixed period of time with 30 μl of quenching solution (Table 2b). This solution normally contains 140 mM KCl and 1 mM LaCl$_3$, which effectively stops the transvesicular movement of Ca^{2+}. A 220-μl aliquot from the total of 280 μl in the tube is removed, and the vesicles are harvested on 0.45 μm nitrocellulose filters.

TABLE 1
Na$^+$-Ca^{2+} Exchange Reaction Medium Composition (μl per tube)

(Ca^{2+}) (mM)	Na or K	Ca stock (mM)		^{45}Ca	Valino- mycin	DDW	SL	nmol Ca per tube
		0.25	1.0					
5	125	5	—	20	5	90	5	1.25
10	125	10	—	20	5	85	5	2.50
15	125	15	—	20	5	80	5	3.75
20	125	20	—	20	5	75	5	5.00
30	125	30	—	20	5	65	5	7.50
40	125	40	—	20	5	55	5	10.00
50	125	50	—	20	5	45	5	12.50
100	125	—	25	20	5	70	5	25.00
140	125	—	35	20	5	60	5	35.00
160	125	—	40	20	5	55	5	40.00
200	125	—	50	20	5	45	5	50.00

Solutions for Reaction Media

Table 1a   K$^+$ or Na$^+$ Diluting Solution (pH = 7.4 at 37°C)

	MW	mM	100 ml	250 ml	500 ml
NaCl	58.44	280	1.64 g	4.09 g	8.18 g
KCl	74.6	280	2.09 g	5.22 g	10.44 g
MOPS	209.3	20	0.418 g	1.046 g	2.093 g

Table 1b   Ca^{2+} Stock Solution

	MW	mM	25 ml	50 ml	100 ml
CaCl$_2$	147.02	100	0.368 g	0.735 g	1.470 g

Note: From this stock solution make two working stock solutions of 0.25 and 1.0 mM.

Table 1c   Valinomycin Stock Solution

	MW	mM	25 ml	50 ml	100 ml
Valinomycin	1111.4	80	2.22 mg	4.45 mg	8.89 mg

Note: Bring to volume with absolute ethanol and store at 4°C. Just prior to experiment, take an aliquot and dilute 1:4 with H$_2$O to generate a working stock solution. A positive displacement pipette works well for this aliquot. Typically for these experiments, 100 μl of the valinomycin stock is diluted with 300 μl H$_2$O. Add 5 μl of the working stock solution to each tube, which results in final concentrations of 0.4 μM valinomycin and 0.5% EtOH.

Table 1d ^{45}Ca^{2+} Stock Solution and Standard

^{45}Ca^{2+} can be ordered with a radioactivity of 20 mC$_i$/ml and a specific radioactivity of 15 to 30 mCi/mg. From this, a 50-μl aliquot is withdrawn and diluted with 50 ml of DDW to give a stock solution with a radioactivity of 20 μCi /ml and is kept at 4°C. 20 μl of this stock solution is added to each tube, making the radioactivity and the added Ca^{2+} to be ~400 nCi and 0.1 to 0.3 nmol, respectively, per tube. The standard for this experiment is taken from any of the tubes at the end of the experiment. Each tube has a total volume of 280 μl after the quenching and 60 μl after the 220-μl aliquot is removed for filtration. If the ^{45}Ca^{2+} has not decayed substantially, a 20-μl aliquot from any tube should contain ~30 nCi or ~64,000 dpm. The 20-μl aliquot to be considered a standard is applied to an entire filter that is held with forceps by the edge and is not under filtration, keeping all radioactivity on the filter. Normally three samples are used as the standard, and each filter is placed in a separate vial, dried, and counted as above.

TABLE 2

Solutions for Na$^+$-Ca^{2+} Exchange

Table 2a   Sarcolemmal Na$^+$ Loading Solution

	MW	mM	100 ml	250 ml	500 ml
NaCl	58.44	140	0.82 g	2.05 g	4.09 g
MOPS	209.3	20	0.418 g	1.046 g	2.093 g

Table 2b   Quenching/Rinsing Solution

	MW	mM	100 ml	250 ml	500 ml
KCl	74.6	140	1.044 g	2.61 g	5.22 g
LaCl$_3$	371.4	1	37 mg	93 mg	186 mg

Notes: *With reconstituted vesicles, which generally have smaller diameters, normally 0.22-μm filters are used.*

For this procedure we use a Millipore 25-mm fritted glass filter support which is inserted into a silicone stopper, which in turn is placed in a 125-ml filtration flask under vacuum. A 15-ml funnel is clamped to the filter support to allow for vesicle washings. The filters are washed with 3 ml of a rinsing solution (Table 2b) applied through the funnel twice. This solution must be isotonic with the vesicles in order that vesicular rupture does not occur and also it should result in significant removal of Ca^{2+} from the surface of the vesicles to improve the signal-to-noise ratio. The filter is carefully removed with forceps and placed on the bottom of a scintillation vial. The filters are then dried in the vials either for several hours to overnight in a fume hood or about 1 h in an oven set at 50 to 60°C if glass scintillation vials are used. The vials are then filled with 10 ml of scintillation cocktail, mixed and counted by standard liquid scintillation techniques.

2.3. Time Dependence

It is important in these experiments to determine the time dependence of sodium-dependent Ca uptake first in order to establish the period in which initial rates of uptake are occurring. Because of the relatively small vesicular volumes and high rates of transport, the period of initial rates is relatively short. Typically, in our hands, the rates become nonlinear within 3 to 4 seconds; thus it is imperative to determine the Ca^{2+} uptake using reaction times that are less than this if one wishes to determine K_m and V_{max}. Normally 1 to 2 s is appropriate. In order to determine rates over this short a period of time, the reaction can be quenched at fixed and precise intervals using a rapid uptake device (RUD), as shown in Figure 1. The original instrument was designed and built at the Cardiovascular Research Laboratories at UCLA as conceived by K.D. Philipson. The unit shown in Figure 1 is a second generation unit built at Simon Fraser University and thus is referred to as "Son of RUD." This device allows a solenoid to be activated at times ranging from 0.5 to 20 s (chosen by the experimenter by use of a dial setting on the unit) after activation of the reaction. Reactions longer than this can easily be quenched by pipetting by hand. The tubes can be incubated in a water bath at the appropriate temperature until immediately prior to the reaction initiation. The reaction is initiated by a modified vortex unit in which the depression of the rubber tube holder that activates the vortex action also sends a signal to the RUD. This allows the solenoid to be activated at the preset time after reaction initiation. The solenoid causes rapid ejection of a predetermined volume (30 µl) of quenching solution from the Eppendorf repeater pipette into the reaction tubes, thereby stopping the reaction.

While it is not uncommon to report Na^+-Ca^{2+} exchange from periods ranging from initial rates all the way to those of the steady state (~2 min), the later are probably not physiologically relevant. The vesicular calcium content at this time interval reflects a balance of Ca^{2+} influx and efflux from the vesicles. The efflux, in turn, is determined by the intravesicular Ca^{2+} concentration and vesicular permeability to Ca^{2+}. Both of these terms are affected to a large degree by experimental artifacts (vesicular volume and degree of leakiness) over which the experimenter has no control. Thus higher or lower steady state Ca^{2+} vesicular content between two groups may not reflect differences in transport rates and are therefore difficult to interpret.

2.4. Ca^{2+} Concentration Dependence

Once an appropriate time frame is established for determination of initial rates, the $K_m(Ca^{2+})$ and V_{max} can be determined by varying $[Ca^{2+}]_o$ in the reaction tubes as described in Table 1. Typically in this type of experiments, the $K_m(Ca^{2+})$ falls in the range of 10 to 40 μM and, as a consequence, a $[Ca^{2+}]_o$ range of 5 to 200 μM is adequate. However, it should be noted that in the making of these solutions, even if HPLC-grade water is used, the

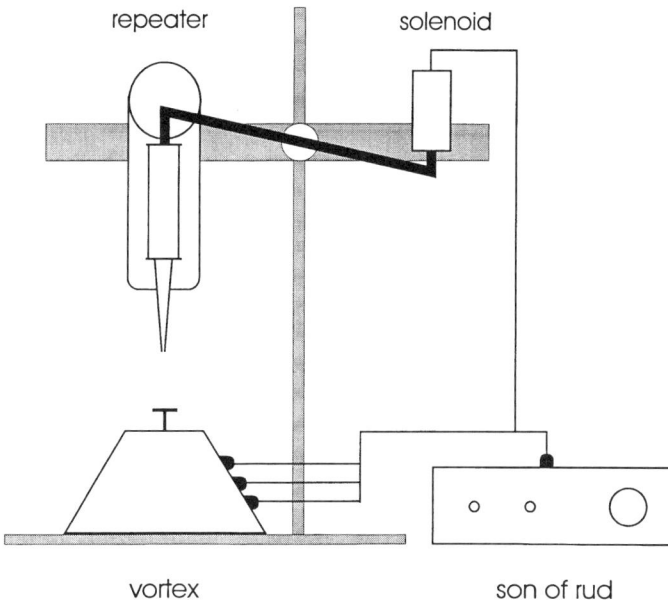

Figure 1
The "Son of RUD" refers to the second generation RUD or rapid uptake device that has been designed for reproducibly quenching the Na$^+$-dependent Ca^{2+} uptake at the short intervals required for initial rate measurements. The RUD activates a solenoid at a preset time to control the ejection of the quenching solution into the reaction tube. The vortex is used both to initiate the reaction as described in the text and to send a signal to the RUD to initiate timing.

co.taminating Ca^{2+} levels are in the low micromolar range. Thus, at the lower values of [Ca^{2+}]$_o$, this error can be significant and should be recognized. Use of Ca^{2+} buffers (e.g., EGTA) to control [Ca^{2+}]$_o$ is not recommended because these buffers can have a direct effect on exchanger activity.[13]

2.5. Passive Efflux

The rate of passive efflux of Ca^{2+} from isolated vesicles may be of some importance in the interpretation of experiments measuring the rates of Na$^+$-Ca^{2+} exchange in cardiac sarcolemmal vesicles from two populations. In order to set up the efflux, it is crucial to load maximally the vesicles with ^{45}Ca^{2+}, which can be done actively or passively. Active loading can best be done on Na$^+$-loaded vesicles and running the Na$^+$-Ca^{2+} exchange reaction for a minimum of 2 min at 37°C as described in the previous section. Alternatively, the vesicles can be passively loaded by letting vesicles incubate overnight at 4°C (or for several hours at room temperature) with a solution containing appropriate amounts of ^{45}Ca^{2+}. A small aliquot can be taken after the loading to determine vesicular Ca^{2+} content prior to initiation of efflux by using the filtration procedure described above.

The efflux is initiated by diluting the solution containing the Ca^{2+}-loaded vesicles five-fold with a solution that will (1) establish an outward directed Ca^{2+} gradient, (2) maintain tonicity to circumvent osmotic shock of the vesicles, and (3) not encourage Ca^{2+} depletion of the vesicles by routes other than passive efflux (e.g., Na^+-Ca^{2+} exchange). Normally a solution of 140 mM KCl and 1 mM EGTA will be appropriate for this assay. If the loading is established by Na^+-Ca^{2+} exchange as described above in Section 2.2, then this dilution used to initiate efflux will result in the following final concentrations in mM: KCl 140, NaCl 0.5 and EGTA 0.8. Under these conditions and assuming the efflux is carried out at 37°C, the extravesicular pCa nominally is 9.2 and should establish an outward directed Ca^{2+} gradient that is more than four orders of magnitude. For the rates of efflux, aliquots are taken at appropriate time intervals (we have used 2, 4, and 6 min) and the Ca^{2+} content at these times are determined by filtering and washing the vesicles as described above.

2.6. Calculations

2.6.1. Worksheet

We use a Microsoft Excel spreadsheet for all of the calculations that are derived from these determinations of ^{45}Ca content. Once the template is set up and the data are entered, all the calculations are performed automatically and the results can be displayed clearly and consistently for each sample. An example of the spreadsheet output using Muscrat cardiac sarcolemma as starting material is shown in Figure 2. From the display of this worksheet and a description of the calculations to be made (as described below), it should be relatively straightforward to construct a worksheet tailored to your applications.

Notes: *If you do not have this capability, you can send a blank PC-formatted 3.5" floppy disk and SASE to the address on the first page; the templates can be sent to you.*

The data to be entered include: (1) the counts from the K^+ and Na^+ diluted vesicles and the standard (which is determined as described above), (2) the protein concentration of the sample, (3) the volumes of the SL and standard aliquots, and (4) the reaction time. From these data, the rates of uptake in nmol/mg SL protein per second at each $[Ca^{2+}]_o$ can be calculated and are used in the plotting of the Eadie Hostee relationship. These two relationships are displayed on our worksheet for each experiment. From this plot, both the V_{max} and the K_m (Ca^{2+}) can be determined.

DATE	06-Dec-95	STD	37885	38219	AVG	38009				STD	20 μl
PREP	Muscrat 1	[Prot]	1.59 mg/ml		37922					SL Vol	3 μl

[Ca] μM	t sec	Ca amt nmol	K1 cpm	K2 cpm	K AVG cpm	Na1 cpm	Na2 cpm	Na AVG cpm	K-Na cpm	nmol /mg	nmol /mg/s	rate/ [Ca]	Est rate
5	2.0	0.089	3378	3221	3300	554	499	527	2773	1.74	0.87	0.17	1.91
10	2.0	0.179	3356	3416	3386	490	474	482	2905	3.64	1.82	0.18	1.55
20	2.0	0.357	3003	3023	3013	463	454	459	2555	6.40	3.20	0.16	2.49
40	2.0	0.714	2197	2232	2215	390	391	390	1824	9.15	4.57	0.11	4.46
100	2.0	1.786	1444	1414	1429	371	345	358	1072	13.43	6.72	0.07	6.49
200	2.0	3.571	990	951	971	375	373	374	597	14.96	7.48	0.04	7.77

Na/Ca X (plot: Uptake (nmol/mg/s) vs [Ca²⁺] μM)

Eadie-Hofstee Plot (Uptake (nmol/mg/s) vs Rate / [Ca²⁺])

EH Plot Estimates:

V_{max}	9.37	nmol/mg/s	K_m	42.96	μM	R^2	0.95

Figure 2

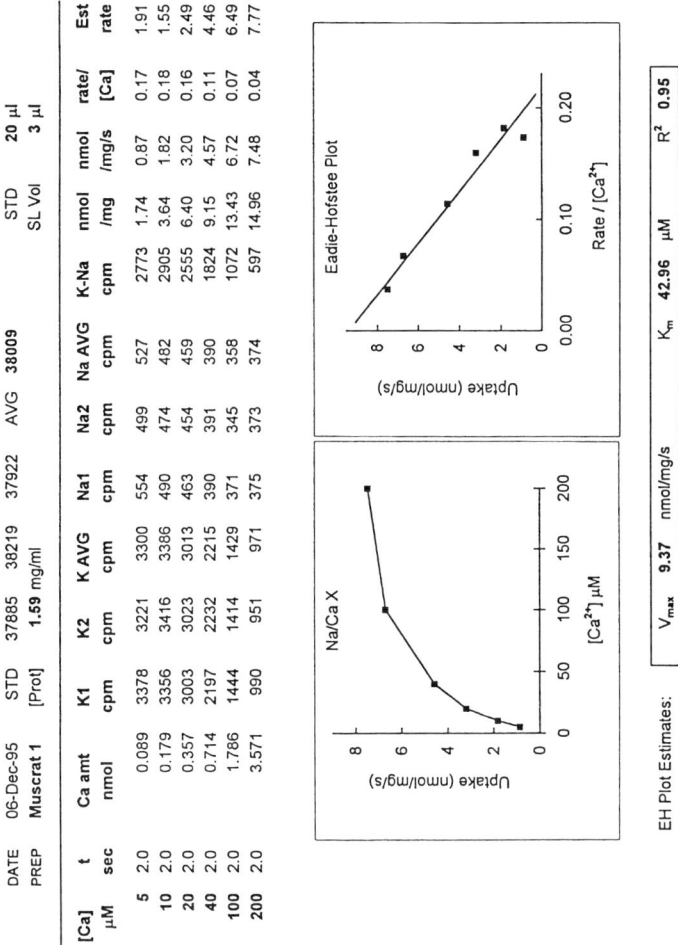

Spreadsheet output sample using Muscrat cardiac sarcolemma as starting material.

3. Conclusions

The radioisotopic measurement of Na$^+$-Ca^{2+} exchange in purified sarcolemmal vesicles is described in this chapter. This technique measures the initial velocities of Na$^+$-dependent uptake of ^{45}Ca^{2+} into vesicles in order that the V$_{max}$ of transport and the K$_m$ (Ca^{2+}) can be accurately assessed. This technique affords one the capability of determining if pathological (e.g., diabetes, pressure overload or ischemia) or physiological (e.g., developmental, exercise, diet, or aging) perturbations affect either the density of exchangers or the affinity of the exchanger for Ca^{2+}. However, the limitations of the procedure must be considered carefully in light of the specific application, and these are discussed in some detail in the chapter.

Acknowledgments

The author gratefully acknowledges grant support from the Heart and Stroke Foundation of British Columbia and Yukon and NSERC of Canada.

References

1. Bers, D.M. and Bridge, J.H.B., Relaxation of rabbit ventricular muscle by Na-Ca exchange and sarcoplasmic reticulum calcium pump, *Circ. Res.,* 65, 334–342, 1989.
2. Bersohn, M.M., Philipson, K.D., and Fukushima, J.Y., Sodium-calcium exchange and sarcolemmal enzymes in ischemic rabbit hearts, *Am. J. Physiol.,* 242, C288–295, 1982.
3. Bersohn, M.M., Vemuri, R., Schuil, D.S., Weiss, R.S., and Philipson, K.D., Effect of temperature on Na$^+$-Ca^{2+} exchange in sarcolemma from mammalian and amphibian hearts, *Biochim. Biophys. Acta,* 1062, 19–23, 1991.
4. Bridge, J.H.B., Spitzer, K.W., and Ershler, P.R., Relaxation of isolated ventricular cardiomyocytes by a voltage-dependent process, *Science,* 241, 823–825, 1988.
5. DiPolo, R., The sodium-calcium exchange in intact cells, in *Sodium-Calcium Exchange,* Allen, T.J.A., Noble, D., and Reuter, H., Eds., Oxford University Press, Oxford, 1989, 5–26.
6. Fabiato, A., Calcium-induced release of calcium from the cardiac sarcoplasmic reticulum, *Am. J. Physiol.,* 245, C1–C14, 1983.
7. Hilgemann, D.W., Regulation and deregulation of cardiac Na$^+$-Ca^{2+} exchange in giant excised sarcolemmal patches, *Nature,* 344, 242–245, 1990.
8. Khananshvili, D., Distinction between the two basic mechanisms of cation transport in the cardiac Na$^+$-Ca^{2+} exchange system, *Biochemistry,* 29, 2437–2442, 1990.
9. Leblanc, N. and Hume, J.R., Sodium-current-induced release of calcium from cardiac sarcoplasmic reticulum, *Science,* 248, 372–376, 1990.

10. Li, Z., Nicoll, D.A., Collins, A., Hilgemann, D.W., Filoteo, A.G., Penniston, J.T., Weiss, J.N., Tomich, J.M., and Philipson, K.D., Identification of a peptide inhibitor of the cardiac sarcolemmal Na+-Ca2+ exchanger, *J. Biol. Chem.*, 266, 1014–1020, 1991.

11. Nicoll, D.A., Longoni, S., and Philipson, K.D., Molecular cloning and functional expression of the cardiac sarcolemmal Na+-Ca2+ exchanger, *Science,* 250, 562–565, 1990.

12. Philipson, K.D., Bersohn, M.M., and Nishimoto, A.Y., Effects of pH in Na+-Ca2+ exchange in canine cardiac sarcolemmal vesicles, *Circ. Res.*, 50, 287–293, 1982.

13. Philipson, K.D. and Nicoll, D.A., Molecular and kinetic aspects of sodium-calcium exchange, *Int. Rev. Cytol.,* 137, 199, 1993.

14. Philipson, K.D., Nicoll, D.A., and Li, Z., The cardiac sodium-calcium exchanger, in *Molecular Biology and Function of Carrier Proteins*, Rockefeller Press, New York, 1993, 188–191.

15. Philipson, K.D. and Nishimoto, A.Y., Stimulation of Na+-Ca2+ exchange in cardiac sarcolemmal vesicles by proteinase pretreatment, *Am. J. Physiol.,* 243, C191–C195, 1982.

16. Reeves, J.P., Bailey, C.A., and Hale, C., Redox modification of sodium-calcium exchange activity in cardiac sarcolemmal vesicles, *J. Biol. Chem.*, 261, 4948–4955, 1986.

17. Reeves, J.P. and Hale, C.C., The stoichiometry of the cardiac sodium-calcium exchange system, *J. Biol. Chem.*, 259, 7733–7739, 1984.

18. Reeves, J.P. and Philipson, K.D., Sodium-calcium exchange activity in plasma membrane vesicles, in *Sodium-Calcium Exchange*, Allen, T.J.A., Noble, D., and Reuter, H., Eds., Oxford University Press, Oxford, 1989, 27–53.

19. Reeves, J.P. and Sutko, J.L., Sodium-calcium exchange in cardiac sarcolemmal vesicles, *Proc. Natl. Acad. Sci. U.S.A.,* 76, 590–594, 1979.

20. Reuter, H. and Seitz, N., The dependence of calcium efflux from cardiac muscle on temperature and external ion composition, *J. Physiol.*, 195, 451-470, 1968.

21. Shi, Z.Q., Davison, A.J., and Tibbits, G.F., Effects of active oxygen generated by DTT/Fe2+ on cardiac Na+/Ca2+ exchange and membrane permeability to Ca2+, *J. Mol. Cell. Cardiol.,* 21, 1009–1016, 1989.

22. Tibbits, G.F. and Philipson, K.D., Na+-dependent alkaline earth metal uptake in cardiac sarcolemmal vesicles, *Biochim. Biophys. Acta,* 817, 327–332, 1985.

23. Tibbits, G.F., Philipson, K.D., and Kashihara, H., Characterization of myocardial Na+-Ca2+ exchange in rainbow trout, *Am. J. Physiol.,* 262, C411–C417, 1992.

24. Vemuri, R. and Philipson, K.D., Phospholipid composition modulates the Na+-Ca2+ exchange activity of cardiac sarcolemma in reconstituted vesicles, *Biochim. Biophys. Acta,* 937, 258–268, 1988.

Chapter **4**

Measurement of Sodium/Potassium ATPase in Myocardium

Vijayan Elimban, Anton Lukas, and
Naranjan S. Dhalla

Contents

1. Introduction 46
2. Measurement of Na$^+$-K$^+$ ATPase Activity 46
   2.1. General Consideration 46
   2.2. Membrane Vesicles and Detergent Treatment 47
   2.3. Na$^+$-K$^+$ ATPase Assay 49
   2.4. Coupled Enzyme Assay 51
3. Measurement of K$^+$-Dependent Phosphatase Activity 53
   3.1. K$^+$-p-Nitrophenyl Phosphatase Activity 53
   3.2. Fluorometric Measurement of K$^+$-Phosphatase Activity 54
4. Measurement of Ouabain Binding to Na$^+$-K$^+$ ATPase 55
5. Applications of the Technique 57
6. Summary 58
Acknowledgments 58
References 58

1.   Introduction

Sodium potassium (Na[+]-K[+]) ATPase is an enzyme present in the plasma membrane of all eukaryotic cells. Since its discovery in 1957 by Skou,[1] this enzyme has been the interest of many investigators. For cardiologists and cardiovascular scientists, this cell membrane protein, which is an enzymatic representation of the Na[+]-K[+] pump, is of particular interest because of its regulatory role in both the excitation and contraction of the heart. Moreover, Na[+]-K[+] ATPase is regarded as the digitalis receptor, and its inhibition is related to both the positive inotropic and toxic effects of cardiac glycosides. There are excellent reviews in the literature about the basic structure, mechanism of action, and regulation of this enzyme pump.[2-5] For any enzyme, proper measurement of its activity is one of the most important aspects of its study. Because of the complex nature of Na[+]-K[+] ATPase, a number of methods are available for its measurement and from time to time these methods have been reviewed by several investigators.[6,7] The aim of this chapter is to provide concise information about the measurement of Na[+]-K[+] ATPase from the heart.

2.   Measurement of Na[+]-K[+] ATPase Activity

2.1.   General Consideration

Although Na[+]-K[+] ATPase facilitates the coupled transport of Na[+] and K[+], the substrate for the enzyme is ATP. Therefore, the most convenient way of measuring enzyme activity is to follow the hydrolysis of ATP by the enzyme. Full activation of this enzyme requires the simultaneous presence of Mg^{2+} and both Na[+] and K[+]. Although K[+] can be replaced by Rb[+], Na[+] cannot be replaced by any other cations.[8] Several partial reactions of the entire Na[+]-K[+] ATPase cycle can be monitored under ideal conditions.[9-16] Among these, Na[+],Mg^{2+}-dependent phosphorylation, which determines the number of active Na[+]-K[+] ATPase molecules, and K[+]-dependent phosphatase activity are convenient determinations to measure enzyme activity. These measurements employ broken cell membranes that consist of either tissue homogenates or purified membrane preparations. Various methods for the isolation of sarcolemmal membranes are discussed elsewhere.[17] The purity of sarcolemmal preparations is assessed by using marker enzyme activities.[17] Although transport of cations does not occur in broken membranes, reconstitution experiments with purified Na[+]-K[+] ATPase indicate that the enzyme activity is identical with the Na[+]-K[+] pump.[18] Usually, pump activity is measured as the ouabain-sensitive ATP hydrolysis. Since ouabain is a specific inhibitor of the Na[+]-K[+] pump, the contribution of other ATPases to the total detected ATP hydrolysis is eliminated by its use. Although vanadate is not a specific inhibitor of Na[+]-K[+] ATPase, this agent is also often used because of its high potency for the enzyme.

The slow rate of interaction between ouabain and Na^+-K^+ ATPase sometimes leads to an overestimation of Mg^{2+} ATPase[19] in the initial stage of
reaction after the addition of ATP. Immediate and complete inhibition of Na^+-
K^+ ATPase is obtained when the concentration of ouabain is at least 1000
times the K_d value. Ouabain concentrations 10 and 100 times the K_d value can
result in approximately 91 and 99% inhibition of the enzyme.[19] This is particularly important for the enzyme from dog or frog heart, since it has relatively
low affinity for ouabain. Normally 1 to 2 mM ouabain is used when the rat
heart enzyme is assayed. Another problem in the use of ouabain arises from
the vesicular nature of the membrane preparations. All membrane preparations
contain a mixture of both "inside-out" and "right-side out" vesicles.[20] Ouabain
is a water-soluble glycoside, and its binding sites to the enzyme are on the
outside of the membrane. Thus, ouabain may not be able bind to "inside-out"
vesicles, so this would yield incorrect information about the enzyme activity.
This problem can be avoided by using either a lipid-soluble glycoside such as
digitoxigenin,[21] or by using substances like alamethicin,[21-24] which makes pores
in the membrane so that ouabain can enter the vesicles. Alternatively, certain
detergents like deoxycholate (DOC) and sodium dodecyl sulfate (SDS)[21-25] can
be used at concentrations which only allow partial solubilization of the membrane. At lower concentrations of the detergent, the Na^+-K^+ ATPase is dissolved
in a fully active $(\alpha\beta)_2$ form, whereas at higher concentrations the enzyme
dissociates into a labile $(\alpha\beta)$ structure.[8] Therefore detergents should be used
carefully because they can solubilize the Na^+-K^+ ATPase into an inactive
enzyme.

2.2.   Membrane Vesicles and Detergent Treatment

As mentioned earlier, membrane preparations are vesicular in nature and can
form either "inside-out" or "right-side out" vesicles depending upon the
method of preparation.[20] Accordingly, the sensitivity to ouabain can differ with
respect to the method of membrane preparation. Ouabain inhibits about 80%
of the Na^+-K^+ ATPase activity in sarcolemmal preparation obtained by LiBr
treatment.[20] On the other hand, only about 15% of the Na^+-K^+ ATPase is
sensitive to ouabain in sarcolemma prepared using the sucrose density gradient
method.[26] Therefore, it is believed that the former sarcolemmal preparation
contains predominantly "right-side out" (about 80% "right-side out" or leaky
and 20% "inside out") vesicles and the latter contains mostly "inside-out"
(85% "inside-out" and 15% "right-side out" or leaky) vesicles. Pretreatment
of sarcolemmal preparations with DOC (0.2 mg/mg protein) rendered the Na^+-
K^+ ATPase from both membrane preparations completely sensitive to ouabain
(Table 1).[20] Similarly, pretreatment of microsomal preparations with SDS (0.3
mg/ml) made both Na^+ plus K^+ stimulated and K^+-phosphatase activities completely sensitive to ouabain, although Mg^{2+} ATPase activity remained inhibited
by about 80%.[23] Therefore, it is a common practice to use different detergents
at low concentrations to unmask the latent Na^+-K^+ ATPase activity. Such

TABLE 1
Effect of Deoxycholate Treatment on Heart Sarcolemma Isolated by Two Different Procedures

Enzyme	Sarcolemma 1		Sarcolemma 2	
	−DOC	+DOC	−DOC	+DOC
Na⁺-K⁺-ATPase (μmol Pi/mg/h)	13.2 ± 0.81	16.5 ± 0.87	17.75 ± 3.7	19.95 ± 2.91
Ouabain-sensitive Na⁺-K⁺-ATPase (%)	80 ± 3	95 ± 2	10 ± 1	97 ± 2

Note: Ouabain sensitivity is tested in the presence of 2 mM ouabain and is expressed as the % inhibition of the Na⁺-K⁺ ATPase. Deoxycholate treatment was carried out at 30°C for 10 min at DOC/protein ratio of 0.2. Sarcolemma 1 and Sarcolemma 2 were prepared by LiBr treatment procedure[22] and sucrose density gradient procedure,[26] respectively. The data in this Table are based on a report from our laboratory.[20]

unmasking causes only a slight destruction of membrane integrity, so that Na⁺, ATP, and ouabain can passively permeate into the membrane vesicles. In support of this concept, 0.3 mg SDS/ml solubilized 50% of the total protein of the membrane, yet almost all the enzyme activity remained in the particulate fraction.[23] Higher concentrations of SDS can inhibit the Na⁺-K⁺ ATPase and this inhibition is related to both SDS and protein concentrations.[27] Therefore, it is important to determine the proper concentration of the detergent to be used to unmask the latent ATPase activity and the same detergent-to-protein ratio should be used when the experiments are repeated.

Alamethicin, by virtue of its membrane perturbing property, is also used to unmask the latent Na⁺-K⁺ ATPase activity.[24] The effect of this amphipathic molecule on the membrane is quantitatively similar to that reported for SDS and DOC on the sarcolemmal enzyme.[23,28] An alamethicin-to-protein ratio of one showed maximum levels of ouabain-sensitive Na⁺-K⁺ ATPase in rat sarcolemmal vesicles, although it depressed both Na⁺-K⁺-stimulated ATPase and basal ATPase activities.[21] It should be pointed out that alamethicin is normally dissolved in alcohol at a very high concentration, but the final alcohol concentration used in the assay mixture should not exceed 0.5%. When SDS and DOC are used, the membrane vesicles should be pretreated with these detergents. Higher concentrations of SDS and DOC markedly inhibit the enzyme activity,[23] so it is necessary to keep the amount of detergent in the final reaction mixture to a minimum. This is achieved either by great dilution or by total removal of the detergents by centrifugation and resuspension.[22,23] Several investigators prefer the latter procedure, as it separates the membranes from the detergent and avoids any further inhibition of the enzyme due to continued contact of detergent with membranes. Apart from this, it offers the flexibility to start the enzyme assay at a later time. DOC treatment of sarcolemmal membrane is done by suspending vesicles in 50 mM Tris-HCl, pH 7.4, containing the detergent at various final concentrations.[22,25] A DOC concentration of 0.2 mg/mg sarcolemma is recommended since this concentration does not

TABLE 2
Composition of Na⁺-K⁺-ATPase Assay Medium

Reagents	Concentration		Volume (μl)			
	Stock (mM)	Final (mM)	Blank	Mg^{2+} ATPase	Na$^+$-K$^+$ ATPase	Ouabain-insensitive Na$^+$-K$^+$ ATPase
NaCl	1,000	100	0	0	100	100
KCl	150	15	0	0	100	100
MgCl$_2$	40	4	0	100	100	100
Tris-HCl (pH 7.4)	500	50	100	100	100	100
Tris-ATP	40	4	100	100	100	100
NaN$_3$	50	5	100	100	100	100
EGTA-Tris	10	1	100	100	100	100
Ouabain	20	2	0	0	0	100
H$_2$O			500	400	200	100
Na$^+$-K$^+$ ATPase (Sarcolemma)	0.25 mg/ml	25 μg/ml	100	100	100	100

inhibit the Mg^{2+} ATPase activity.[25] After mixing, samples are incubated for 10 min at 30°C and the reaction mixture is terminated by the addition of 20 volumes of 1 mM Tris-HCl, pH 7.4. The samples are then centrifuged, washed once, and resuspended in the same buffer. In the case of SDS, pretreatment of membrane is done similarly. Membrane preparations thus obtained are used fresh or small aliquots (5 to 10 mg/ml) are frozen in liquid nitrogen for future use and stored at –80°C without loss of activity for several days. The enzyme activity is more stable when frozen in 0.25 M sucrose and 10 mM histidine (pH 7.4) instead of 50 mM Tris-HCl (pH 7.4). Thawed samples should not be frozen again for future use.

2.3. Na⁺-K⁺ ATPase Assay

The most common assay procedure for Na$^+$-K$^+$ ATPase is the measurement of inorganic phosphate (Pi) released from ATP by the concomitant interaction of Na$^+$, K$^+$, and ATP with the enzyme. A typical reaction mixture for heart sarcolemmal enzyme is shown in Table 2. Briefly, sarcolemmal vesicles (25 μg) are preincubated for 5 min at 37°C in a medium containing 100 mM NaCl, 15 mM KCl, 5 mM MgCl$_2$, 1 mM ethylene glycol-bis (β-aminoethyl ether)-N-N-N'-N'-tetraacetic acid (EGTA), 5 mM NaN$_3$, 2 mM ouabain, and 50 mM Tris-HCl (pH 7.4) in a total volume of 900 μl. To avoid repeated pipetting, the required volumes of common reagents like EGTA, NaN$_3$, and Tris-HCl can be mixed in a beaker and pipetted as a single solution. Stock solution (20 mM) of ouabain is made in water and can be stored in a brown bottle at room temperature for 1 week. As ouabain is light sensitive, it is advised to cover the water bath during incubation. The reaction is started by addition of 100 µl of 40 mM Tris-ATP (Sigma Chemical Co., St. Louis, MO), pH 7.4 (final concentration 4 mM). ATP can be stored frozen as aliquots and used only once after thawing. Na$_2$ATP can also be used in place of Tris-ATP. ATP should be free of vanadate as it is a potent inhibitor of Na$^+$-K$^+$ ATPase. After 10 min, the reaction is stopped by the addition of 1 ml of ice-cold 20% trichloroacetic acid (TCA). The mixture is centrifuged at 4°C (1000 g) for 5 min to remove the precipitated protein, and 0.5 ml of the supernatant is used for estimation of the Pi liberation by the enzyme reaction. Several methods are available for the estimation of Pi in the supernatant.[29,30] All the methods yield equally good results, providing a calibration curve is constructed each time using a 50 to 200 µmol KH$_2$PO$_4$ standard solution. According to the method of Taussky and Shorr,[30] the "blank" tube contains 1.5 ml 12% TCA. "Standard" tubes are made with 1.45 ml 12% TCA and 0.05 ml solution containing 50 to 200 µmol KH$_2$PO$_4$. The "experimental" tube contains 1.0 ml of 12% TCA and 0.5 ml of the supernatant, as mentioned earlier. Add 1 ml of freshly prepared ammonium molybdate-FeSO$_4$ solution. In order to prepare this solution, 1.25 g FeSO$_4$ is dissolved in 22.5 ml water and 2.5 ml 10% ammonium molybdate (dissolved in 10 N H$_2$SO$_4$) is slowly added. Ammonium molybdate solution can be prepared and stored in a brown bottle for several weeks. The color is measured after 10 min at 693 nm. The amount of phosphate is calculated from the standard curve. If the protein concentration is very low (5 µg), centrifugation can be avoided without any interference on the Pi estimation. This information is important, as ATP is unstable at acidic pH. Therefore, the estimation of Pi should be completed as quickly as possible. ATP hydrolysis at acidic pH is minimized at low temperature; therefore the centrifugation should be done only at 4°C. This situation is avoided if the ATPase reaction is followed by the production of ATP rather than Pi (see Section 2.4). Membrane protein concentration is estimated by the method of Lowry et al.[31] Enzyme activity is usually expressed as µmol Pi/mg protein/h. Parallel experiments are done either with Na$^+$ + K$^+$ + ouabain or with Mg^{2+} + ouabain omitted from the reaction medium. Na$^+$-K$^+$ ATPase is calculated as the difference between the activity registered with and without Na$^+$ plus K$^+$ in the absence of ouabain. The difference in enzyme activity calculated in the absence and presence of ouabain gives the ouabain-sensitive Na$^+$-K$^+$ ATPase.

The pH optimum for the reaction is about 7.4, but any pH in the range of 6.9 to 7.4 can be used without an appreciable loss of activity.[32,33] With the broken membrane preparation, the optimal activity is measurable at 130 mM Na$^+$ and 20 mM K$^+$, and the Na$^+$/K$^+$ ratio that gives optimal activity is about 6.5. Slight changes in the concentration of these cations do not make any appreciable difference in activity.[34] Because the K$_m$ value for Na$^+$-K$^+$ ATPase is very high, ATP at a concentration of 3 mM or more is routinely used; 1 mM free Mg^{2+} yields maximal activity. ADP exerts an inhibitory effect on Na$^+$-K$^+$ ATPase, so the concentration of ADP should be kept to about 10 to 15% of the ATP concentration during the reaction. It is important to keep the time of incubation in a linear range so that ADP is not accumulated above this level. Normally 10 min incubation is recommended. The ADP concentration can also be reduced by using phosphoenol pyruvate (PEP) (Sigma Chemical Co.)/pyruvate kinase (PK) (Sigma Chemical Co.)[21] as an ATP-regnerating system. The inclusion of PEP/PK in the assay medium is also recommended if the ATP concentration is very low once the K_m value for the enzyme is determined; 2.5 mM PEP and 10 IU/ml PK are routinely added to the reaction mixture.

Caution: *Tris buffer counteracts the effect of K^+ and should thus be used with caution.*

Since Tris-HCl is a very efficient buffer at pH 7.4, it is the choice of many investigators. Imidazole-HCl or histidine-HCl can also be used at this pH range. Histidine buffer can not be used in studies that test the effect of free radicals on Na^+-K^+ ATPase, since it is a scavenger. Glycerol, which is used as a preservative for protein, also inhibits Na^+-K^+ ATPase and should be kept below 5%.[32] This also holds true for sucrose and DMSO. Na^+-K^+ ATPase measurement in sarcolemma can be affected by other ATPases present in the sarcolemmal membrane and by contamination from mitochondria and sarcoplasmic reticulum when tissue homogenates are used. Inclusion of 1 mM EGTA in the reaction mixture eliminates the influence by SR and SL Ca^{2+}-stimulated ATPases. Mitochondrial ATPase is inhibited by 5 mM NaN_3, which possibly inhibits the regeneration of ATP from ADP and Pi by mitochondria.

2.4.   Coupled Enzyme Assay

Na^+-K^+ ATPase can also be assayed by measuring ADP produced during the reaction using a coupled enzyme system containing auxiliary enzymes.[35] The mathematical models and analysis of coupled enzyme systems are discussed by Rudolph et al.[36] The ADP produced by the Na^+-K^+ ATPase reaction is monitored from the oxidation of NADH in the presence of phosphoenol pyruvate (PEP) and two auxiliary enzymes, namely, pyruvate kinase (PK) and lactate dehydrogenase (LDH), as shown below.

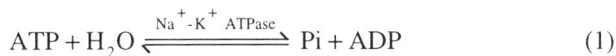

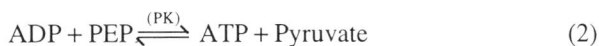

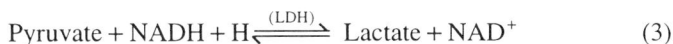

$$ATP + H_2O \overset{Na^+\text{-}K^+ \text{ ATPase}}{\rightleftharpoons} Pi + ADP \tag{1}$$

$$ADP + PEP \overset{(PK)}{\rightleftharpoons} ATP + Pyruvate \tag{2}$$

$$Pyruvate + NADH + H \overset{(LDH)}{\rightleftharpoons} Lactate + NAD^+ \tag{3}$$

The reaction mixture contains all the ingredients mentioned in the measurement of Pi release (see above), as well as 0.2 mM NADH (Boehringer Mannheim), 2.5 mM PEP (Boehringer Mannheim), 10 U/ml PK (Boehringer
Mannheim) and 30 U/ml LDH (Boehringer Mannheim). The total volume of
reaction mixture used is 3 ml. Aliquots of the stock solutions are pipetted into
glass or quartz cuvettes of 1-cm light path and placed into the temperature-
controlled cuvette compartment of the spectrophotometer and equilibrated to
37°C. A cuvette containing distilled water is placed in the reference compartment. The reaction is initiated by the addition of membrane suspension. The
reaction mixture is stirred well with a plastic rod or pipette tip, and the enzyme
activity is recorded automatically at 340 nm. A chart depicting various steps
in this method is given in Figure 1. Decrease in absorbance of NADH per min
(ΔA) is estimated and the Na$^+$-K$^+$ ATPase activity is calculated from the molar
extinction coefficient of NADH (6.22×10^3 cm$^{-1} \cdot$ M^{-1}).

$$\frac{\text{Specific activity of}}{\text{Na}^+\text{-K}^+ \text{ ATPase}} = \frac{\Delta A \times (\text{vol. of assay, in ml}) \times 10^6}{6.22 \times 10^3 \times (\text{mg protein used for assay}) \times 10^3}$$

$$= \mu\text{mol ADP/mg protein/min}$$

The ouabain-sensitive Na$^+$-K$^+$ ATPase activity is obtained as the difference
between activities in the absence and presence of ouabain. The advantage of
this method is the ability to continuously monitor the reaction. As a steady
level of ATP is maintained by a constant conversion of ADP, the inhibitory
effect of ADP on the enzyme is also eliminated. One of the drawbacks of this
assay procedure is the difficulty of estimating the Mg^{2+}-ATPase activity. As
pyruvate kinase activity requires K$^+$, the ATPase reaction can not be measured
in the absence of K$^+$. Very high concentrations of ouabain (in the order of
1000 times the K$_d$ value) can be used to inhibit Na$^+$-K$^+$ ATPase for this purpose.
It is possible that the ATP in the assay mixture is contaminated with ADP (1
to 2%), which can oxidize some of the NADH and bring down the A$_{340}$ for
0.2 mM NADH to 0.8 to 0.9 from the theoretical value of 1.25.[35] The practical
upper limit for Na$^+$-K$^+$ ATPase concentration in the assay is about 0.1 U/ml
by this method, and therefore the enzyme protein concentration selected should
be kept to a minimum. Because of the continuous monitoring of the reaction,
it is advantageous to use this method to monitor the reaction kinetics of various
compounds on the Na$^+$-K$^+$ ATPase activity, provided these compounds do not
affect the PK and LDH in the reaction mixture.

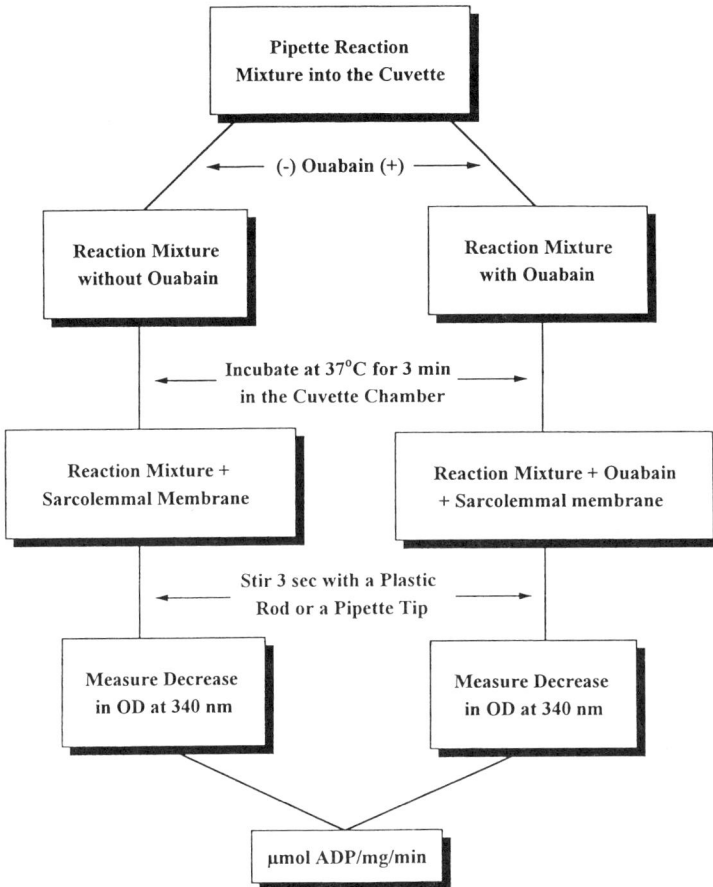

Figure 1
Different steps involved in the enzyme-coupled assay for the determination of Na+-K+ ATPase. The reaction mixture contains ingredients listed in Table 2 as well as 0.2 mM NADH, 2.5 mM PEP, 10 U/ml PK and 30 U/ml LDH. The total volume of the reaction mixture is 3 ml. Sarcolemmal proteins are 50 mg, whereas the concentration of ouabain is 2 mM.

3. Measurement of K+-Dependent Phosphatase Activity

3.1. K+-p-Nitrophenyl Phosphatase Activity

Na+-K+ ATPase activity can be measured indirectly by following the dephosphorylation step of the reaction.[32] The enzyme can hydrolyze several phosphatase-type substrates like acetyl phosphate, p-nitrophenyl phosphate (pNPP), carbonyl phosphate, and methyl fluorescein phosphate in the presence of Mg^{2+}. The reaction does not require Na^+ and the most commonly used substrate is pNPP. K^+-dependent p-nitrophenyl phosphatase activity is measured[37] in 50 mM Tris-HCl, pH 7.8, 5 mM MgCl$_2$, 1 mM EGTA, 5 mM pNPP (Sigma Chemical Co.) and 20 mM KCl at 37°C. The reaction volume is 1 ml and contains 8 μg of sarcolemmal protein. The K^+-independent phosphatase activity measured in the absence of K^+ is subtracted. The reaction is quenched after 10 min with 2 ml of 1 N NaOH, and the absorbance at 410 nm is used to determine the amount of p-nitrophenol formed. At high pH, p-nitrophenol is intense yellow. The absorption peak of p-nitrophenol is below 410 nm, and this wavelength is chosen to eliminate interference from pNPP. A standard curve with various p-nitrophenol (Sigma Chemical Co.) concentrations (0.025 to 0.1 mM) is used to calculate the p-nitrophenol formed.

Ouabain is not an effective inhibitor of K^+-pNPPase. Therefore, the use of ouabain can overestimate the basal activity and underestimate the K^+-stimulated reaction velocity. Tris and choline counteract the effect of K^+; glycerol increases the K^+-pNPPase activity, in contrast to its effect on Na^+-K^+ ATPase activity.[35] The K^+-pNPPase activity, is 5- to 7-fold lower than the Na^+-K^+ ATPase; however, the procedure is very sensitive, due to the high absorption intensity of the final product formed (p-nitrophenol), which makes it possible to use low enzyme concentrations. Another advantage of this assay procedure is the low background absorbance. This method can not be used for continuous measurement of enzyme activity because the reaction is terminated with NaOH in order to measure p-nitrophenol concentration.

3.2. Fluorometric Measurement of K^+-Phosphatase Activity

3-O-Methyl fluorescein phosphate (MFP) is used as the substrate[6,38] for the K^+-phosphatase assay method described by Huang and Askari.[16] The incubation conditions are very similar to those described for K^+-pNPPase above except that MFP (Sigma Chemical Co.) is used as substrate instead of p-nitrophenol phosphate. Enzyme preparations are incubated with 1 mM MgCl$_2$ and 50 mM Tris-HCl, pH 7.5, with or without 10 ml KCl in a temperature-controled sample chamber of a spectrofluorometer maintained at 37°C. After 5 min preincubation, the reaction is started by the addition of MFP (final concentration 10 or 20 μM). The product 3-O-methyl fluorescein formed is recorded continuously (excitation maximum 475 nm and emission maximum 525 nm). The fluorometer is always standardized with a solution of 3-O-methyl fluorescein (Sigma Chemical Co.) in the same buffer as used for the assay. A stock standard solution (2 mM) is prepared in methanol and can be stored in the freezer. This solution is diluted (1:100) with 50 mM NaOH and is stored in the refrigerator. A further dilution (1:200) with distilled water is necessary to give the highest working standard. The procedure can be used for enzyme kinetic studies because of the ability to continuously record the reaction by this method. Fluorometric analysis is very sensitive, and it is emphasized that highest purity reagents, fresh water, and thoroughly clean glassware must be used.

4. Measurement of Ouabain Binding to Na+-K+ ATPase

There are a number of factors that influence the binding of cardiac glycosides to Na+-K+ ATPase.[11,39,40] Although Na+-K+ ATPase isolated from different sources has similar affinities for ligands such as Na+, K+, Mg^{2+}, and ATP, the affinity for cardiac glycosides varies widely in enzyme preparations from different sources and within a single species. This led to the discovery of different molecular forms of Na+-K+ ATPase with low and high affinities for cardiac glycosides from different tissues.[41,42] Another factor that influences the binding affinity is the chemical structure of the cardiac glycoside used. [^{3}H]-ouabain is widely used by many investigators, primarily because of its high water solubility. This allows the preparation of high stock solution without using organic solvents, which often inhibit the enzyme activity. Moreover, ouabain has very low nonspecific binding, and this provides a more precise estimation of the enzyme concentration compared to the assay of phosphory-lated intermediates.

The specific binding of [^{3}H]-ouabain can be used to assess Na+-K+ ATPase in membrane preparations and to measure the number of active pump sites in the intact cells. Matsui and Schwartz[43] suggested that digitalis binds to a phosphorylated conformation of Na+-K+ ATPase which requires Mg^{2+} and ATP and is stimulated by Na+ and depressed by K+. This binding can also take place in the presence of Mg^{2+} and Pi, but under this condition both Na+ and K+ are known to inhibit the binding.[44] These two situations are called type I and type II conditions, respectively, because the enzyme–inhibitor complexes formed under these conditions are different.[45] Since the addition of Mg^{2+} increases the affinity of ouabain by several fold, both type I and type II conditions are ideal for binding studies.[46] However, Mg–Pi-supported ouabain binding is strongly inhibited by high ionic strength so the concentration of buffer should be 10 mM under this assay condition.

To determine high and low affinity [^{3}H]-ouabain binding in sarcolemmal preparations,[21] 35 μg membrane protein is incubated in a reaction mixture containing 1.5 mM MgCl$_2$, 1.0 mM phosphate (inorganic phosphate titrated to pH 7.5 with Tris), 10 mM Tris-HCl, pH 7.5 at 37°C and 0 to 5000 nM [^{3}H]-ouabain (specific activity 4.42 Ci/mmol; diluted from the stock). Determinations are performed in the absence or presence of 2.0 mM ouabain, a concentration sufficient to inhibit >95% of the specific [^{3}H]-ouabain binding. SDS (9 μg/ml) is added directly to the assay mixture to permeabilize the sarcolem-mal vesicles to ouabain. The reaction is started by the addition of [^{3}H] ouabain and terminated after 1 h by filtration (Millipore, HAWP 25 mm, 0.45 μm) using a Millipore filtration unit. Filters are washed three times with 2.5 ml ice-cold washing solution containing 10 mM Tris-HCl, pH 7.5, 0.1 mM oua-bain and 15 mM KCl. Filters are normally presoaked with washing solution for 30 min. The type of filter does not make a difference in the binding studies except that pore size should be 0.45 μm. Filters with larger pore size (0.8 μm) may allow passage of small membrane fragments. On the other hand, a smaller pore size (0.2 μm) may clog the filters and reduce the filtration rate to cause dissociation of the bound ligands. This can also occur with 0.45 μm filters when higher amounts of membrane proteins are used. Filters are dissolved and counted for radioactivity by standard procedure. The nonspecific [^{3}H]-ouabain binding is obtained in the presence of excess ouabain. The data on [^{3}H]-ouabain binding is analyzed using the LIGAND computer program.[47,48] Dissociation constant (K_d) and maximal density (B_{max}) for low and high affinity binding sites for ouabain with Na$^+$-K$^+$ ATPase are obtained from a Scatchard plot (Figure 2).

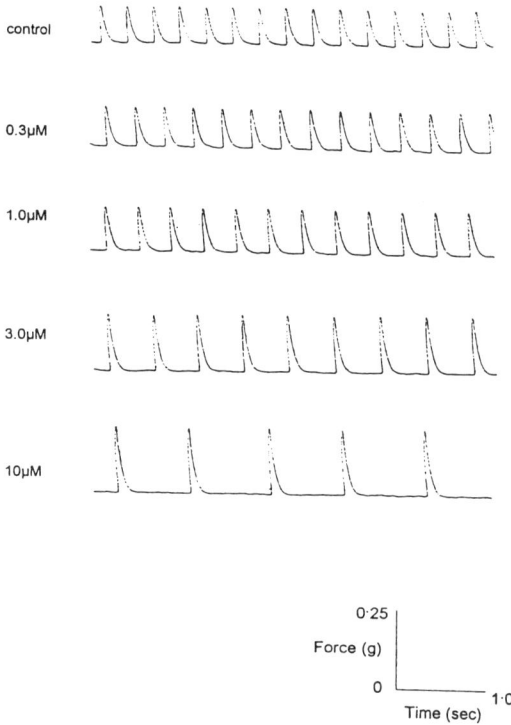

Figure 2

Scatchard plot analysis of data on specific binding on [^{3}H]-ouabain with cardiac sarcolemmal membranes. Results with low concentrations of [^{3}H]-ouabain indicating high affinity site are given in the inset, whereas those with high concentrations of [^{3}H]-ouabain indicating low affinity site are given in the main figure. These results on specific binding were obtained by using 1 to 5000 nM [^{3}H]-ouabain (specific activity 4.42 Ci/mmol).

Ouabain binding can also be performed in a medium containing 100 mM NaCl, 5 mM MgCl$_2$, 5 mM Tris-ATP, and 50 mM Tris-HCl. This condition is better suited for leaky vesicles since neither ATP nor [^{3}H]-ouabain can enter intact vesicles. As heart sarcolemmal and microsomal preparations typically contain both intact and leaky vesicles, the binding in this medium requires the pretreatment of membranes with detergents. In contrast, binding in the presence of Mg^{2+} + Pi occurs in both leaky and intact vesicles and is recommended for membrane preparations.

[^{3}H]-ouabain is obtained from New England Nuclear (Boston, MA) and usually has a specific activity of about 15 Ci/mmol and purity of about 99%. The rate of decomposition is about 1% for 6 months, and under ideal storage conditions, it can be used for several months. It is reported that the specific radioactivity of the commercial preparation may be different from the value given by the supplier.[49] This may give different ouabain concentrations in the reaction mixture than the calculated value. Therefore it is necessary to estimate the exact concentration of ouabain in each batch of [^{3}H]-ouabain.[49] A simple spectrophotometric method[50] is discussed by Wallick and Schwartz for this purpose. In order to get a good Scatchard plot, 10 to 90% occupation of receptors should be obtained.[50] The values obtained at equilibrium of the binding reaction should be used for this purpose. In enzyme preparations with low affinity for ouabain, the equilibrium may be reached faster in comparison to ouabain-sensitive preparations, which may require at least 90 min incubation time. Therefore it is necessary to determine the time required to reach binding equilibrium. When sarcolemmal preparations or homogenates are used, the binding reaction may level off as a result of ATP depletion and ADP formation. Under these circumstances, Mg–Pi-dependent binding condition are particularly useful.

5.   Applications of the Technique

The Na^+-K^+ ATPase directly or indirectly contributes to the regulation and maintenance of many cellular processes, including cell volume, $[pH]_i$, $[Ca^{2+}]_i$, and resting membrane potential. In turn, numerous ionic and hormonal influences on the cell regulate the activity of this essential enzyme. Thus, a simple assay to accurately measure Na^+-K^+ ATPase activity has many potential useful applications. The measurement of Na^+-K^+ ATPase activity provides a means to study the mechanisms of action of drugs that alter the excitation–contraction coupling process in the myocardium by affecting Na^+-pump mechanisms. In drug screening, a Na^+-K^+ ATPase assay system can identify potential new inotropic agents that exert their effect through inhibition of the sodium pump in addition to gaining information regarding their potencies. Since the therapeutic window of cardiac glycosides is rather low and continuous use of these agents leads to arrhythmia, such an assay system can screen new drugs to predict potentially arrhythmogenic side effects due to inhibition of the sodium pump. The assay to determine Na^+-K^+ ATPase activity presented in this chapter is also applicable in the study of the pathophysiology of heart dysfunction. Changes in Na^+-K^+ ATPase activity and/or ouabain binding sites occur in such diverse pathophysiological conditions as heart failure, ventricular hypertrophy, myocardial ischemia, myocardial infarction, and aging heart. Thus, the ability to monitor Na$^+$-K$^+$ ATPase activity can provide important information about the mechanisms underlying these disease states as well as the beneficial effects of certain cardiac drugs.

6. Summary

This chapter discusses the methods for the measurement of cardiac Na$^+$-K$^+$ ATPase activity. Problems associated with techniques for monitoring the enzyme activity in membrane preparations are identified. Biochemical and fluorometric methods for the measurement of K$^+$-p-nitrophenyl phosphatase and K$^+$-phosphatase, which represent dephosphorylation steps of the Na$^+$-K$^+$ ATPase reaction, have been outlined, respectively. The measurement of [^{3}H]-ouabain binding, which represents another index of the Na$^+$-K$^+$ ATPase activity has also been outlined. It is hoped that this article will serve as a useful reference source for investigators engaged in studying the status of Na$^+$-K$^+$ ATPase in myocardium in health and disease.

Acknowledgments

The research work reported in this article was supported by a grant from the Medical Research Council of Canada (MRC Group in Experimental Cardiology). Dr. Lukas is the Myles Robinson Scholar.

References

1. Skou, J. C., The influence of some cations on an adenosine triphosphatase from peripheral nerves, *Biochim. Biophys. Acta,* 23, 394, 1957.
2. Bonting, S. L., Sodium-potassium activated adenosine triphosphatase and cation transport, in *Membrane and Ion Transport,* Bittar, E. E., Ed., Wiley Interscience, London, 1970, chap. 8.
3. Baker, P. F., Blaustein, M. P., Keynes, R. D., Mani, J., Shaw, T. I., and Steinhardt, R. A., The ouabain sensitive fluxes of sodium and potassium in squid giant axon, *J. Physiol. (London),* 459, 1969.
4. Eisner, D. A. and Smith, W., The Na$^+$-K$^+$ pump and its effectors in cardiac muscle, in *The Heart and Cardiovascular System,* Fozzard, H. A., Jennings, B. R., Haber, E., and Katz, A. M., Eds., Raven Press, New York, 1992, chap. 35.
5. Fozzard, H. A. and Gunn, R. B., Membrane transport, in *The Heart and Cardiovascular System,* Fozzard, H. A., Jennings, B. R., Haber, E., and Katz, A. M., Eds., Raven Press, New York, 1992, chap. 6.

6. Akera, T., Methods for studying digitalis receptors, Na^+-K^+ ATPase and sodium pump activity in heart membrane and myocardium, in *Methods in Studying Cardiac Membrane*, vol. 2, Dhalla, N. S., Ed., CRC Press, Boca Raton, FL, 1984, chap. 11.

7. Fleischer S. and Fleischer, B., Eds., *Methods in Enzymology*, vol. 156, Academic Press, San Diego, CA, 1988.

8. Skou, J. C., The Na^+-K^+ pump, *News Physiol. Sci.*, 7, 95, 1992.

9. Albers, R. W., Biochemical aspects of active transport, *Annu. Rev. Biochem.*, 36, 727, 1967.

10. Post, R. L., Kume, S., Tobin, T., Orcutt, B., and Sen, A. K., Flexibility of an active centre in sodium-potassium adenosine triphosphatase, *J. Gen. Physiol.*, 54, 306S, 1969.

11. Thomas, R., Gray, P., and Andrews, J., Digitalis: its mode of action, receptor and structure-activity relationship, *Adv. Drug Res.*, 19, 311, 1990.

12. Fahn, S., Koval, G. J., and Albers, R. W., Sodium-potassium-activated adenosine triphosphatase of electrophorus electric organ. I. An associated sodium-activated transphosphorylation, *J. Biol. Chem.*, 241, 1882, 1966.

13. Fahn, S., Hurley, M. R., Koval, G. J., and Albers, R. W., Sodium-potassium activated adenosine triphosphate of electrophorus electric organ. II. Effect of N-ethyl maleimide and other sulfhydryl reagents, *J. Biol. Chem.*, 241, 1890, 1966.

14. Albers, R. W., Fahn, S., and Koval, G. J., The role of sodium ions in the activation of electrophorus electric organ adenosine triphosphatase, *Proc. Natl. Acad. Sci. U.S.A.*, 50, 474, 1963.

15. Ahemed, K. and Judah, J. D., Preparation of lipoproteins containing cation-dependent ATPase, *Biochim. Biophys. Acta*, 93, 603, 1964.

16. Huang, W. and Askari, A., (Na^+-K^+)-activated adenosine triphosphatase. Fluorometric determinations of the associated K^+-dependent 3-O-methyl fluorescein phosphatase and its use for the assay of enzyme samples with low activities, *Anal. Biochem.*, 66, 265, 1975.

17. Dhalla, N. S. and Pierce, G. N., Isolation and characterization of the sarcolemmal membrane from the heart, in *Methods of Studying Cardiac Membrane*, vol. 1, Dhalla, N. S., Ed., CRC Press, Boca Raton, FL, 1984, chap. 1.

18. Skou, J. C., Enzymatic basis for active transport of Na^+ and K^+ across cell membrane, *Physiol. Rev.*, 45, 596, 1965.

19. Akera, T., Quantitative aspects of interaction between ouabain and (Na^+-K^+) ATPase in vitro, *Biochim. Biophys. Acta*, 249, 53, 1971.

20. Moffat, M. P., Singal, P. K., and Dhalla, N. S., Differences in sarcolemmal preparations. Cell surface material and membrane sidedness, *Basic Res. Cardiol.*, 78, 451, 1983.

21. Dixon, I. M. C., Hata, T., and Dhalla, N. S., Sarcolemmal Na^+-K^+ ATPase activity in congestive heart failure due to myocardial infarction, *Am. J. Physiol.*, 262, C664, 1992.

22. Pierce, G. N. and Dhalla, N. S., Sarcolemmal Na^+-K^+ ATPase activity in diabetic heart, *Am. J. Physiol.*, 245, C241, 1983.

23. Besch, H. R., Jones, J. R., and Watanabe, A. M., Intact vesicles of canine cardiac sarcolemma. Evidence from vectoral properties of Na$^+$-K$^+$ ATPase, *Circ. Res.,* 39, 586, 1976.

24. Jones, L. R., Maddock, S. W., and Besch, H. R., Unmasking effect of alamethicin with Na$^+$-K$^+$ ATPase, β-adrenergic receptor-coupled adenylate cyclase and cAMP-dependent protein kinase activities of cardiac sarcolemmal vesicles, *J. Biol. Chem.,* 255, 9971, 1980.

25. Panagia, V., Lamers, J. M., Singal, P. K., and Dhalla, N. S., Ca^{2+}- and Mg^{2+}- dependent ATPase activities in the deoxycholate-treated rat heart sarcolemma, *Int. J. Biochem.,* 14, 387, 1982.

26. Kidwai, A. M., Radcliffe, M. A., Dunchon, G., and Daniel, E. E., Isolation of plasma membranes from cardiac muscle, *Biochem. Biophys. Res. Commun.,* 45, 901, 1971.

27. Jorgenson, P. L., Purification of Na$^+$/K$^+$ ATPase: enzyme source, preparative problems and preparation from mammalian kidney, *Methods Enzymol.,* 156, 29, 1988.

28. Seppet, E. K. and Dhalla, N. S., Characterization of Ca^{2+}-stimulated ATPase in rat heart sarcolemma in the presence of dithiothreitol and alamethicin, *Mol. Cell Biochem.,* 91, 137, 1989.

29. Fiske, C. H. and Subbarow, Y., The colorimetric determination of phosphorus, *J. Biol. Chem.,* 66, 375, 1975.

30. Taussky, H. and Shorr, E., A microcolorimetric method for the estimation of inorganic phosphorus, *J. Biol. Chem.,* 202, 678, 1953.

31. Lowry, O. H., Rosebrough, N. J., Farr, A. L., and Randal, R. J., Protein measurement with Folin phenol reagent, *J. Biol. Chem.,* 193, 265, 1951.

32. Esmann, M., ATPase and phosphatase activity of Na$^+$,K$^+$ ATPase: molar and specific activity, protein determination, *Methods Enzymol.,* 156, 105, 1988.

33. Sulakhe, P. V., Elimban, V., and Dhalla, N. S., Characterization of a partially purified Na$^+$-K$^+$ ATPase from dog heart, in *Adv. Myocardiol.,* Dhalla, N. S. and Hearse, D. J., Eds., Plenum Publishing, 1985, 6, 249.

34. Skou, J. C., Effect of ATP on the intermediary steps of the reaction of the (Na$^+$-K$^+$) ATPase. IV. Effect of ATP on K$_D$s for Na$^+$ and on hydrolysis at different pH and temperature, *Biochim. Biophys. Acta,* 567, 421, 1979.

35. Norby, J. G., Coupled assay of Na$^+$-K$^+$ ATPase activity, *Methods Enzymol.,* 156, 116, 1988.

36. Rudolph, F. W., Bangher, B. W., and Beissner, R. S., Techniques in coupled enzyme assays, *Methods Enzymol.,* 63, 22, 1979.

37. Kutryk, M. J. B. and Pierce, G. N., Stimulation of sodium-calcium exchange by cholesterol incorporation into isolated cardiac sarcolemmal vesicles, *J. Biol. Chem.,* 263, 13167, 1988.

38. Drapeau, P. and Blostein, R., Interactions of K$^+$ with (Na$^+$,K$^+$) ATPase, *J. Biol. Chem.,* 255, 7827, 1980.

39. Schwartz, A., Lindenmeyer, G. E., and Allen, J. C., The sodium-potassium adenosine triphosphatase: pharmacological, physiological and biochemical aspects, *J. Pharmacol. Rev.,* 27, 1, 1975.

40. Hansen, O., Interactions of cardiac glycosides with ($Na^+ + K^+$)-activated ATPase. A biochemical link to digitalis induced ionotropy, *Pharmacol. Rev.,* 36, 143, 1984.

41. Lindenmayer, G. E. and Wellsmith, N. V., Two receptor forms for ouabain in sarcolemma-enriched preparations from canine ventricle, *Circ. Res.,* 47, 710, 1980.

42. Ng, Y. C. and Akera, T., Two classes of ouabain binding sites in ferret heart and two forms of Na^+-K^+ ATPase, *Am. J. Physiol.,* 252, H1016, 1987.

43. Matsui, H. and Schwartz, A., Mechanism of cardiac glycoside inhibition of ($Na^+ + K^+$)-dependent ATPase from cardiac tissue, *Biochim. Biophys. Acta,* 151, 685, 1968.

44. Schwartz, A., Matsui, H., and Laughter, A. H., Titrated digoxin binding to ($Na^+ + K^+$)-activated adenosine triphosphatase: possible allosteric sites, *Science,* 160, 323, 1968.

45. Akera, T. and Brody, T. M., Membrane adenosine triphosphatase. The effect of potassium on the formation and dissociation of the ouabain enzyme complex, *J. Pharmacol. Exp. Ther.,* 176, 545, 1971.

46. Wallick, E. T., Pitts, B. J. R., Lane, L. K., and Schwartz, A., A kinetic comparison of cardiac glycoside interactions with (Na^+-K^+)-ATPase from skeletal and cardiac muscle, *Arch. Biochem. Biophys.,* 202, 442, 1980.

47. McPherson, G. A., Analysis of radioligand binding experiments. A collection of computer programs for the IBM-PC, *J. Pharmacol. Methods,* 14, 213, 1985.

48. Munson, P. J. and Robbard, D., Ligand: a versatile computerized approach for characterization of ligand binding systems, *Anal. Biochem.,* 107, 220, 1980.

49. Akera, T. and Cheng, V. J. K., A simple method for the determination of affinity and binding site concentrations in receptor binding studies, *Biochim. Biophys. Acta,* 640, 779, 1981.

50. Wallick, E. T. and Schwartz, R. A., Interaction of cardiac glycosides with Na^+-K^+ ATPase, *Methods Enzymol.,* 156, 201, 1988.

Chapter 5

Molecular Assessment of Cardiac Sodium Pump Activity

Vijayan Elimban, Kiminori Kato, and
Naranjan S. Dhalla

Contents

1. Introduction..64
2. Measurement of Sodium Pump Activity in Intact Cells......................65
   2.1. [^{3}H]-Ouabain Binding...65
   2.2. ^{86}Rb$^+$-Uptake 66
3. Measurement of Phosphorylated Intermediates 67
   3.1. Phosphorylation by [γ^{32}P]-ATP 68
   3.2. Phosphorylation by [^{32}P]-Orthophosphate...........................69
4. Measurement of Na$^+$-K$^+$ Pump ATPase Isozymes 70
   4.1. SDS Polyacrylamide Gel Electrophoresis and Western Blot
        Analysis...72
   4.2. Isolation of mRNA and Northern Blot Analysis........................73
5. Summary 77
Acknowledgments...78
References...78

0-8493-3333-4/97/$0.00+$.50

1. Introduction

Sodium-potassium ATPase is considered a marker enzyme for the cell membrane and is known to hydrolyze ATP on the cytosolic face of membranes during transport of 3 Na^+ per ATP to the extracellular fluid in exchange for 2 K^+.[1] This coupled transport is electrogenic in nature, with a net positive charge transported out per cycle, and, thus, contributes significantly to maintenance of transmembrane potential. Under physiological conditions this exchange is about 200 cycles per second.[2] According to the Albers-Post model,[3,4] the Na^+-K^+ ATPase exists in a number of conformational states during the reaction cycle (Figure 1). The model basically shows that the Na^+-K^+ ATPase catalyzes a Na^+-dependent phosphorylation followed by a K^+-dependent dephosphorylation. The enzyme has a regulatory site that binds cardiac glycosides and contributes to their inhibitory effect on the Na^+-K^+ pump activity.[5]

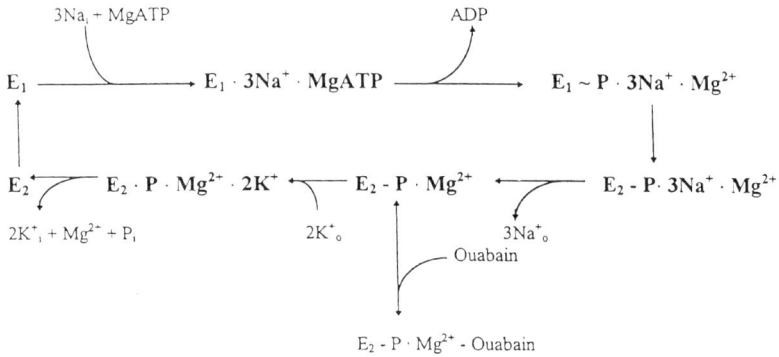

Figure 1

Modified version of the Albers-Post model of Na^+-K^+ ATPase reaction. E_1, E_2, E_1~P, and E_2-P are major conformational states of Na^+-K^+ ATPase during the reaction cycle. Subscripts i and o denote inside and outside, respectively.

The Na^+-K^+ ATPase consists of two polypeptides, namely, the α and β subunits.[1] The α subunit has a molecular mass of about 112 kDa and has catalytic activity. The β subunit is required for the enzyme activity, but no specific function has been attributed to this 35-kDa protein. The molar ratio of α to β is 1:1 in the membrane. Recent work from several laboratories indicates that the α and β subunits exist in different isoforms in human and experimental animals.[6-9] At least three isoforms exist for the α subunit (α_1, α_2, and α_3), and these are detectable at mRNA and protein levels. Three isoforms for the β subunit (β_1, β_2, and β_3) have also been cloned and sequenced.[6,7] The physiological significance of these isozymes remains obscure; however, they differ markedly in their affinity to Na^+ and sensitivity to cardiac glycosides. They are differentially regulated under various physiological and pathological conditions, suggesting unique physiological functions of these isoforms. In this discussion, we focus on the molecular assessment of the sodium pump. Although assessment of the isozymes can be done using specific antibodies, the unique nature of the Na^+-K^+ ATPase pump allows for the measurement of subunit isozymes from the phosphoprotein intermediate formed in the presence of low and high concentrations of ouabain.

2. Measurement of Sodium Pump Activity in Intact Cells

Recent developments in the understanding of cell biology have simplified the measurement of Na^+-K^+ pump activity in intact cells, especially cardiac cells. However, it is important to consider alterations in cellular physiology created by the isolation process when the Na^+-K^+ pump is studied in the intact cell. The method for isolation of intact cardiomyocytes is discussed elsewhere.[10] There are several methods used to provide accurate analysis of Na^+-K^+ pump activity in intact cells. These include measurement of $^{22}Na^+$ efflux,[11] [³H] ouabain binding,[12] ouabain-sensitive $^{86}Rb^+(K^+)$ uptake,[11] and ouabain-sensitive oxygen consumption.[13] Under most circumstances, the measurement of ouabain-sensitive $^{22}Na^+$ efflux is not easy and accurate; therefore $^{86}Rb^+$ uptake is widely used. However, [³H] ouabain binding is the most widely used method to measure Na^+-K^+ pump activity on the cell surface, because the cardiac glycosides bind to the extracellular side of the sodium pump rapidly and dissociate slowly. Therefore these two methods are discussed below.

2.1. [³H]-Ouabain Binding

It is clear that ouabain primarily binds to the phosphorylated intermediate or E_2P configuration of the Na^+-K^+ pump.[14] The enzyme turnover is a prerequisite for binding under normal physiological conditions. The rate-limiting step in the ATPase cycle is the association of Na^+ and ATP with the enzyme (Figure 1). When cells become ATP or Na^+ depleted, the Na^+-K^+ pumps stall in the E_1 configuration and ouabain can not bind to the enzyme. When cells under these conditions are warmed or oxygenated, ATP hydrolysis may resume with subsequent formation of phosphorylated intermediates and ouabain binding.[15,16] From equilibrium binding studies it is possible to estimate the maximum number of Na^+-K^+ pumps per cell at saturating concentrations of the ligand. However, if the ouabain concentration is far below the saturating concentration, such that less than 10% of Na^+-K^+ pumps are bound, the turnover rate of the pump in cell suspension can be obtained. External K^+ inhibits the binding of ouabain to the sodium pump whereas Na^+ promotes ouabain binding. Therefore binding studies should be performed in a K^+-free medium or isotonic buffered saline. Since there are at least two receptor binding sites present on the Na^+-K^+ pump, the binding must be carefully analyzed before reporting the relative population of these receptors.

Cultured heart cells are routinely used to measure the number of Na^+ pump sites on the cell membrane. Most of the studies employ 10-day-old chick heart.[17,18] Monolayer cultures of spontaneously contracting chick embryo ventricular cells are prepared for this purpose.[19,20] About 4 to 5×10^5 cells attached to the petri dish are incubated in a K^+-free buffered solution (pH 7.35) containing 4 mM N-2-hydroxy ethylpiparazine-N'-2 ethane sulfonic acid (HEPES), 0.05 mM $CaCl_2$, 137 mM NaCl, 0.5 mM $MgCl_2$, and various concentrations of [^{3}H] ouabain (62.5 to 2000 nM) for 15 min at 37°C. Stock [^{3}H] ouabain (15.4 Ci/mmol) is diluted to give a specific activity of 7.7 Ci/mmol. Unlabeled ouabain is added to achieve the desired final concentration when necessary. At the end of the incubation, the cells are quickly scraped from the cover slip and filtered through a microfiber filter (Millipore, pore size 0.22 μm). Filters are washed 3 times with ice-cold HEPES buffered solution (pH 7.35) containing 4 mM KCl. Radioactivity on the filters is determined using a liquid scintillation spectrophotometer by standard procedure. The total [^{3}H]-ouabain binding minus the nonspecific binding obtained in the presence of 10^{-3} M unlabeled ouabain gives the specific [^{3}H]-ouabain binding at each [^{3}H]-ouabain concentration.

To measure protein content of cells on each cover slip,[17] they are incubated for 24 h before the experiment with L-[^{14}C(U) Leucine] (0.0005 μCi/ml), which incorporates into the cell protein. Cells on plates not exposed to [^{3}H]-ouabain are washed 3 times for 5 min by placing them in a large volume of cold buffer solution. The cells are dissolved and assayed for protein content by the method of Lowry et al.[21] Accurate estimation of the protein concentration of the cells is obtained from the relationship between ^{14}C and measured protein concentration. Simultaneous counting of ^{14}C and ^{3}H allows the measurement of [^{3}H]- ouabain bound per milligram cell protein. Maximum binding (B_{max}) is used to calculate the pump sites per cell, and the K_d is obtained from Scatchard plot analysis as described earlier.[22,23]

Although the method described above used cells in monolayers, it is possible to adapt the procedure for cells in suspension like adult heart cells. Such a method is described by English and Schultz.[24] Ouabain binding is an excellent method for studying the number of Na^+-K^+ pumps in intact cells; this method is not suitable for rats and mice because of the very high K_d values. This situation makes the quantitation of pump difficult, due to the rapid rate of ouabain dissociation from the pump sites.

2.2. ^{86}Rb$^+$-Uptake

The Na^+-K^+ pump activity in the intact cell can also be determined from the measurement of ouabain-sensitive, unidirectional influx of ^{86}Rb$^+$ which behaves similarly to K^+,[1] and can replace K^+ for influx studies. ^{86}Rb$^+$ is usually used for transport studies because it has a longer half life (18.7 d) than $^{42}K^+$ (12.4 h). A serious problem often encountered during transport studies in the cell membrane is the existence of multiple modes of transport system in parallel. As cardiac glycosides specifically bind to Na^+-K^+ ATPase, the ouabain-sensitive $^{86}Rb^+$ uptake gives an estimate of the ongoing Na^+-K^+ pump activity in the cell without any interference from any other transport activity. When the sodium pump activity is estimated from the ouabain-sensitive $^{86}Rb^+$ or $^{42}K^+$ uptake, it is necessary to evaluate whether the observed activity actually represents the rate of Na^+ efflux. The transport ratio of 3 Na^+ to 2 K^+ may be substantially reduced under conditions in which the amount of Na^+ available to the Na^+-K^+ pump is greatly reduced and the extracellular K^+ is relatively high.[25] Therefore, the use of relatively low concentrations of K^+ (1 mM) or Rb^+ (2 mM) in the incubation mixture is essential.[26] Moreover, the binding of ouabain to Na^+-K^+ ATPase is antagonized by K^+.[27]

For the most part, monolayers of cultured cells are used for uptake ($^{86}Rb^+$ or $^{42}K^+$) studies.[17,28] But the procedure can be modified for cells in suspension.[24] Atrial muscle preparations of guinea pig and rat or ventricular papillary muscle are also used for uptake studies. When monolayers are used, the unbound radioactivity can be washed easily from the cover slip. Cell suspensions have to be centrifuged through oil (silicone oil:dinonyl phthalate, 1:1) in order to isolate cells from the unbound isotopes and to reduce the nonspecific binding.[24]

The rate of $^{86}Rb^+$ uptake can be measured by incubating the cover slip containing 4 to 5×10^5 cells in a K^+-free phosphate-buffered saline (PBS) (150 mM NaCl, 10 mM Tris- phosphate, containing 2 mM RbCl with 2.5 µCi of $^{86}Rb^+$) in the presence and absence of ouabain. The reaction is stopped after 15 min by the aspiration of the assay medium and the cover slip is washed rapidly 4 times with cold (4°C) K^+-free PBS. The cells are scraped from the cover slip and dissolved in 2 ml of 1% SDS. Aliquots are counted in a liquid scintillation spectrophotometer by standard procedure. A small aliquot of the sample is used for protein estimation by the method of Lowry et al.[21] after precipitating by 12% TCA and dissolving in NaOH. The ouabain-sensitive $^{86}Rb^+$ uptake is calculated from the difference between the values obtained in the absence and presence of 1 mM ouabain.

3.   Measurement of Phosphorylated Intermediates

On the basis of tracer exchange experiments, Skou[29] proposed the formation of a high energy phosphate intermediate (acylphosphate) of the enzyme (E~P) during the Na^+-K^+ ATPase reaction cycle. According to his scheme, the sodium ion stimulates the formation of a phosphorylated intermediate from ATP, and the potassium ion stimulates its breakdown. When the assay is conducted in the presence of Na^+ + Mg^{2+} + $[\gamma^{32}P]ATP$, which favors the forward direction of the reaction, phosphorylated intermediate is formed by "front door" phosphorylation.[30] However, due to the presence of several other ATPases in crude membrane preparations, it is often difficult to identify and quantitate the Na^+-pump activity. Alternatively, the reaction can be forced to operate in the reverse direction in the presence of Mg^{2+} and ouabain by using inorganic phosphate. This eliminates phosphorylation from other ATPases.[31,32] The alkali-labile covalent phosphorylated intermediate of the enzyme formed through this "back door" phosphorylation is chemically identical to that formed by ATP phosphorylation.[30,32]

3.1. Phosphorylation by [γ³²P]-ATP

Estimation of phosphorylated intermediates in the presence of Na^+ + Mg^{2+} + ATP provides a rapid estimation of the active Na^+-K^+ pump in the enzyme preparation. When the enzyme preparation is incubated with [γ³²P]ATP, a phosphoenzyme is formed rapidly, even at very low temperatures. A low concentration of ATP is required due to the presence of high affinity catalytic sites. About 25 μg of the enzyme preparation is incubated in the presence of 100 mM NaCl, 1 mM $MgCl_2$, and 50 mM Tris-HCl (pH 7.4) in a final volume of 1 ml at 0°C. The reaction is started by the addition of 0.05 mM [γ³²P]ATP (20 to 50 μCi) and terminated after 5 s by the addition of 4 ml of ice-cold trichloroacetic acid containing 1 mM unlabeled ATP and 1 mM orthophosphoric acid (TAP). Nonspecific binding is similarly measured using a reaction mixture containing 100 mM KCl, 1 mM $MgCl_2$, 0.1 mM Tris-ADP, 0.05 mM [γ³²P]ATP, and 50 mM Tris-HCl (pH 7.4). The reaction mixture is filtered under vacuum through Millipore filters (HAWP, 25 mm, 0.45-μm pore size) using a Millipore filtration unit (catalog no. XX1002530). The filters are washed 2 times with 4 ml of ice-cold washing solution (TAP). The filters are transferred to scintillation vials and dissolved in cytoscint-ES (ICN Biomedical) cocktail, and the radioactivity is estimated using a scintillation spectrophotometer. Nonspecific binding is subtracted from total binding observed in the presence of 100 mM KCl to calculate the amount of phosphorylated intermediates. Accurate estimations are difficult due to high background counts. Under these circumstances, [³H] ouabain binding studies provide a better estimate of the active enzyme. A better quantitation of the active pump under these circumstances can be obtained by "back-door" phosphorylation using [³²P] orthophosphate, discussed later.

Since only the catalytic subunit (α) is phosphorylated during the reaction, this procedure can be used to quantitate the active sodium pump.[33-35] When the phosphorylation reactions are performed in the presence of different concentrations of ouabain (high and low), two molecular forms of the Na^+ pump ($α_1$ and $α_2$; for a discussion of these isoforms, see Section 5.4) can be detected on SDS polyacrylamide gels.[33-35] Quantitation of these bands as a function of ouabain concentration determines the relative abundance of these two molecular forms. The effect of ouabain on phosphoenzyme formation is usually examined using the procedure described by Lytton et al.[35] Membranes (100 to 150 µg) are incubated at 37°C for 45 min in an incubation mixture containing 1 mM MgCl$_2$, 1 mM Tris-phosphate, 25 mM Tris-HCl (pH 7.2), and 0 to 1 mM ouabain in a total volume of 50 µl. The samples are chilled in ice. A 40-µl aliquot of each sample is mixed with 10 µl of a mixture containing 50 µM [γ^{32}P]ATP (20 to 50 µCi) and 500 mM NaCl. The reaction is stopped after 30 s by the addition of 50 µl Laemmli[36] sample buffer containing 125 mM Tris-HCl (pH 6.8), 4% SDS, 20% glycerol, 10% 2-mercapthoethanol, and 0.0075% bromophenol blue. The samples are incubated at 37°C for 10 min, and 50-µl aliquots containing 40 to 60 µg protein are loaded onto SDS-polyacrylamide gels (7.5%). Electrophoresis is performed at 10°C using the method described by Laemmli.[36] Lower temperature increases the stability of acylphosphate under alkaline conditions. However, a very low temperature will precipitate the SDS. To increase the resolution between two closely spaced bands it is often necessary to run the dye front off the bottom of the gel for 1 to 2 h. The gels are stained with Coomassie blue, destained, dried onto two layers of cellophane sheet, and exposed to Kodak X-OMAT X-ray film at −70°C with a Dupont Cronex intensifying screen. Quantitation of phosphorylation is performed by densitometric scanning of the appropriate region of the autoradiogram using model GS-670 Imaging Densitometer (BioRad Laboratories).

Phosphorylated intermediates are relatively unstable under the alkaline conditions of the electrophoresis mentioned above. Because of the poor separation of the two forms of Na$^+$-K$^+$ ATPase in acidic gel, alkaline Laemmli gel is the choice of many investigators.[33] SDS-polyacrylamide gel electrophoresis (SDS-PAGE) can also be performed at acidic pH (4.0) using methylene green as a tracking dye.[37,38]

3.2. Phosphorylation by [^{32}P]-Orthophosphate

The assay procedure for the phosphorylation of Na$^+$-K$^+$ ATPase through the "back door" phosphorylation method has been discussed by Resh[31] and Lytton et al.[35] Membranes (50 to 100 µg) are incubated in 1.5 ml Eppendorf tubes for 1 to 2 h at room temperature in 100 µl of a reaction mixture containing 100 mM HEPES, pH 7.4 with Tris-base, 5 mM MgCl$_2$, and varying concentrations of H$_3$PO$_4$ ranging from 10 to 100 µM in the presence of 0 to 1 mM ouabain. The carrier-free [^{32}Pi] is first diluted with Tris/HEPES/MgCl$_2$ buffer to 1 mCi/ml and filtered through a Millipore Millex-Gs 0.22-µm filter unit to remove phosphate polymers which often cause high background. Phosphorylation is started by the addition of 10 to 20 µl [^{32}Pi] to the reaction medium and incubation for 30 min, which is sufficient for the reaction to reach equilibrium. The reaction is quenched by the addition of 50 µg bovine serum albumin as carrier, followed immediately by 1 ml of ice-cold 20% trichloroacetic acid containing 0.1 M H$_3$PO$_4$ (TCAPi). The tubes are placed on ice for 5 min to form the precipitate and centrifuged in an Eppendorf microfuge for 2 min (10,000 g) and washed 3 times with 1 ml each of TCAPi. The final pellet can be analyzed by gel electrophoresis or dissolved in 0.5 ml 5% SDS by sonication and an aliquot counted in a scintillation counter. The radioactivity present in the samples without ouabain is subtracted from the identical samples containing ouabain to obtain the amount of phosphate incorporated covalently into Na⁺-K⁺ ATPase.[31]

The total number of Na⁺ pumps in the membrane can be calculated from a Lineweaver- Burk plot (1/mol phosphate incorporated vs. 1/phosphate concentration). The reciprocal of the Y intercept represents the maximal phosphorylation capacity. From this number, the Na⁺ pumps per milligram membrane protein are calculated. The reciprocal of the X axis intercept gives the K_m for phosphate. Several additional calculations can be made from the number of Na⁺ pump sites. The turnover number of the enzyme for ATP is obtained by dividing Na⁺-K⁺ ATPase activity by Na⁺ pump sites. Usually this number is in the order of 10,000/site/min at 37°C. The number of Na⁺ pumps per cell can also be calculated if the membrane protein per cell is estimated. Based on the K⁺ uptake (⁸⁶Rb⁺ uptake) and assuming 2 K⁺ transported per ATP hydrolyzed, the turnover number of ATP per intact cell can be calculated. The "back door" phosphorylation can also be used to quantitate α_1 and α_2 isoforms of Na⁺-K⁺ ATPase by starting the phosphorylation at two different concentrations of ouabain; a low concentration of ouabain (3 to 5×10^{-6} M) saturates nearly all α_2 sites and only very few α_1 sites, whereas a high concentration (1 mM) saturates both α_1 and α_2 isoforms with ligand. From these results, it is possible to calculate the number of pumps in the α_1 and α_2 forms.

It is important that only the activity of the Na⁺-K⁺ ATPase is measured under the experimental conditions. This can be assured in several ways.[39] First, the phosphorylation in the absence of ouabain should be less than 10% of the level in the presence of ouabain. Second, 100 mM NaCl should be added to inhibit greater than 80% of the ouabain-dependent phosphorylation. Finally, radiolabel incorporation into the catalytic subunit should be visualized using PAGE followed by autoradiography. The acidic pH PAGE described by Amory et al[40] is recommended for this purpose because the acylphosphate bond is alkali labile.

4. Measurement of Na⁺-K⁺ Pump ATPase Isozymes

It is still debatable whether Na⁺-K⁺ ATPase exists as an α-β protomer or a large assembly of α_2-β_2 dimers. Nonetheless, the existence of two subunits, α and β, is well established. Although early evidence for the existence of multiple forms of Na⁺-K⁺ ATPase came from ouabain binding studies, the first demonstration of two molecular forms of Na⁺-K⁺ ATPase was not possible until the application of high resolution SDS-PAGE.[35,41] It is now well established that multiple forms of both α and β subunits (isozymes) exist for Na⁺-K⁺ ATPase from different species and from different tissues within the same species. Recent reports indicate that the α_3 isoform of the rat has a slightly lower mobility on SDS-PAGE than the α_2 isoform.[42,43] Three isoforms of α subunit, namely α_1, α_2, and α_3 and three isoforms of β subunits, namely, β_1, β_2, and β_3 have been cloned and sequenced.[6-9] Although the exact role of β subunits is not well established, they appear to be required for the Na^+-K^+ ATPase activity. The level of β subunit mRNA is substantially lower than the level of expression of any α subunit mRNAs in adult liver[44] and lung.[7] These differences in the levels of α and β subunit mRNAs suggest that translational or posttranslational mechanisms may serve to maintain equimolar amounts of both subunits of Na^+-K^+ ATPase. It is also suggested that β subunits regulate, through assembly of $\alpha\beta$ heterodimers, the number of sodium pumps transported to the plasma membrane.[45]

The newborn rat heart expresses the α_1 and α_3 isoforms, whereas the adult rat heart expresses α_1 and α_2. There is a developmental transition between α_3 and α_2 during the first 3 weeks of postnatal life,[44,46-48] which has been documented at both mRNA and protein levels. Additionally, atria have less α_2 mRNA than ventricle.[6] Changes in the relative amounts of α isoform mRNA in myocardium occur in hypertension[48] and hypertrophy.[49] Isoform specific changes in various other conditions also have been reported.[45,50-52] Thus it is becoming increasingly important to corroborate the results on enzyme activity with studies on isoenzymes and their expression. Although relative amounts of α and β isoform mRNA can be determined with cDNA probes, relative protein levels of isoform can not be determined with antibodies, as the affinity of these antibodies is highly variable. Moreover, protein levels of isoforms can not be predicted from the mRNA level due to isoform specific translation changes. The level of α subunits expressed in a tissue does not always predict transport and enzyme activity as the $\alpha\beta$ assembly is the functional unit for the enzyme.

The production of antibodies specific to different isoforms of Na^+-K^+ ATPase enables the examination of the expression pattern of these proteins. There are a number of polyclonal (antisera) and monoclonal antibodies raised for one or more forms of Na^+-K^+ ATPase isoforms.[8,53] Polyclonal antibodies raised against one form of Na^+-K^+ ATPase cross-react with other forms to some degree. On the other hand, monoclonal antibodies, although more specific in their reaction, more often recognize only native enzymes or only denatured enzymes. A series of antibodies against rat Na^+-K^+ ATPase isoforms has been developed recently. McK_1 is specific for α_1, which can recognise α_1 isozyme from rat, mouse, human, and monkey but not from other species.[54] McB_2 is specific for α_2 and cross- reacts with all mammalian and chicken α_2 isoforms.[8] $McBX_3$ has the highest affinity for α_3 but weakly cross-reacts with α_1.[8] Polyclonal antibodies to α_1, α_2, α_3, β_1, and β_2 are available from Upstate Biotechnology (Lake Placid, NY).

4.1.   SDS-Polyacrylamide Gel Electrophoresis and Western Blot Analysis

To examine α- and β-isoenzymes of Na⁺-K⁺ ATPase translated into protein, 20 to 50 μg purified membrane or homogenate is electrophoresed by the method of Laemmli,[36] using a 4% stacking gel and 7.5% separating gel. Crude membrane preparations are sometimes used to minimize potential selective enrichment of the isoforms during membrane purification. It is also advisable to use proteolytic inhibitors like phenyl methyl sulfonyl fluoride during membrane preparation to prevent proteolysis. After the addition of Laemmli buffer, the sample is not heated to 100°C, but instead it is incubated for 10 min at 37°C; this procedure prevents blurs. Addition of fresh β-mercaptoethanol to the sample is recommended as oxidized β-mercaptoethanol will also blur the resolution.[33] Prestained marker proteins are simultaneously run as standards. After the electrophoresis, the proteins are horizontally transferred to polyvinylidene difluoride (PVDF) membrane (Immobilon-P, Millipore, Bedford, MA) using a transblot cell (BioRad Laboratories, Mississauga, ON) according to the method of Burnette.[55] The transblot cell is maintained at 10°C during the transfer using a refrigerated waterbath. The transblot cell is connected to a power supply (model 200/2.0; BioRad Lab) and the transfer is run at 0.55 Å for 2.5 h.

Once the transfer is completed, immunoblotting is performed as described by Harris et al.[56] The power is shut off, the sandwich disassembled, and the Immobilon-P membrane washed with 20 mM Tris-HCl, pH 6.8, 137 mM NaCl (TBS). The blots are then blocked in 5% (w/v) nonfat dry milk in TBS (TBS bloto) for 60 min at room temperature. This blocking serves to saturate the nonspecific protein binding sites. The blocking solution is discarded and the blots are then incubated for 60 min at room temperature with specific antisera at the proper dilution in TBS bloto. The dilution of the primary antibodies required to give optimum results will vary and should be standardized with each antibody. Alternately, the blots can be incubated with antibodies in TBS bloto overnight at 4°C. The blots are then washed 3 times for 15 min with TBST (20 mM Tris-HCl, 137 mM NaCl, 0.1% Tween 20) to remove any nonspecifically bound antibodies. Antigen–antibody complexes are visualized by incubating the membrane with 0.1 μCi/ml of ¹²⁵I-protein A in TBST buffer for 1 h at room temperature. The blots are then washed 3 to 5 times with TBST for 15 min each before drying and packing the blots in plastic seal-a-meal bags. Once the Western blot transfer and immunoblotting is completed, the sealed blots are placed face upward between two intensifying screens (Lightning Plus model; Dupont Cronex Co.). An X-OMAT film (Eastman Kodak Co., Rochester, NY) is placed on top of the blot in the dark, and the autoradiographic cassette is then incubated at −70°C. Autoradiograms are developed and scanned with a densitometer to determine the relative intensity of the band.

Bound antibodies can also be detected by the enhanced chemiluminescence (ECL) technique using ECL Western blot kit (Amersham, Oakville, ON). The ECL technique is preferred due to its high sensitivity and nonradioactive nature. Biotinylated antibody or horseradish peroxidase (HRP)-labeled second antibody can be used for this purpose. Due to the sensitivity of the ECL technique, the dilution of the second antibody should be optimized to give the highest signal with minimum background. With HRP-labeled antibody, the suitable starting dilution is 1:1000. The membrane is incubated in diluted antibody for 1 h at room temperature. The membrane is washed 3 times (15 min each) with TBST and then treated with detection reagents (see below). If biotinylated second antibody (1:3000 in TBST) is used after washing the membrane with TBST, it is incubated for 45 to 60 min with diluted (1:5000 in TBST) streptavidin-HRP conjugate, and then the membrane is washed with TBST for 15 min, 3 times. Thorough washing of the membrane reduces the background. The biotinylated antibody technique is more sensitive than HRP-labeled second antibody procedure. For detecting the proteins, incubate the membrane in equal volumes of detection reagents 1 and 2 for 1 min. About 0.125 ml reagent/cm^2 membrane is sufficient. Drain off the excess reagent and wrap the blots between two sheets of transparent membrane and expose the blots on Hyperfilm ECL (Amersham) for 15 to 60 s and develop like normal X-ray film. It is necessary to work quickly once the blots are exposed to the detection solution. In fact, all the steps for detecting the proteins can be carried out in the dark room. The intensity of the bands is measured by densitometry using an imaging densitometer (BioRad Laboratories).

4.2. Isolation of mRNA and Northern Blot Analysis

Several investigators use guanidium salts, inhibitors of ribonuclease, as a deproteinizing agent in the isolation of RNA.[57-59] Chirgwin et al.[58] combined guanidium thiocyanate extraction of the tissue with ultracentrifugation through CsCl for the isolation of RNA. By eliminating the ultracentrifugation step, Chomczynski and Sacchi[59] simplified the procedure and used acid guanidium thiocyanate–phenol–chloroform extraction for the isolation of total RNA. This procedure can be used for the isolation of RNA from large (30 g tissue) or small (3 mg tissue or 10^6 cells) amounts of tissue. A modified method of Chomczynski and Sacchi[59] for the isolation of total RNA is described below.

Procedure

1. Cardiac tissue is quickly removed from the anesthetized rat and immediately frozen in liquid nitrogen and stored at −80°C until use.

2. For 500 mg to 1 g tissue (wet weight), add 1 ml of solution D (4 M guanidinium thiocyanate, 25 mM sodium citrate, pH 7.0; 0.5% sarcosyl; 0.1 M 2-mercaptoethanol) and homogenize for 1 min using a polytron.

3. Add 0.1 ml 2 *M* sodium acetate (pH 4.5), 1 ml water-saturated phenol, and 0.2 ml of a mixture of chloroform-isoamyl alcohol (49:1).

4. Vortex the mixture for 30 s and incubate on ice for 15 min.

5. After centrifugation at 4000 rpm at 4°C for 20 min, transfer the aqueous phase containing RNA to a new tube.

6. Add 1 ml of water-saturated phenol and 0.2 ml of chloroform-isoamyl alcohol mixture.

7. Stir for 10 s and centrifuge at 4000 rpm for 10 min at 4°C.

8. Transfer the aqueous phase to a new tube and add diethyl pyrocarbonate (DEPC)-treated (0.1%) distilled water up to the original volume (1 ml).

9. Add 1 ml of isopropyl alcohol and incubate at –20°C overnight.

10. Centrifuge the samples at 7000 rpm for 30 min at 4°C.

11. The pellet is resuspended in 75% ethanol and centrifuged at 7000 rpm for 15 min at 4°C.

12. Discard the supernatant and to the pellet add 300 µl of 0.3 *M* sodium acetate (pH 7.0) and 900 µl of 100% ethanol.

13. Keep the sample at –70°C.

14. A small aliquot is diluted with DEPC-treated water, and the absorbance values at 260 and 280 nm are measured and the ratio (260/280) is calculated. A value close to 2 is indicative of the RNA purity. The concentration of RNA is estimated from the absorbance at 260 nm using the formula,

$$\text{RNA } (\mu g/ml) = \text{Abs}_{260nm} \times \text{dilution factor} \times 40$$

The total RNA content of the tissue can be calculated from the weight of the sample used for RNA preparation.

15. The RNA samples are separated electrophoretically according to the method described by Lehrach et al.[60] using a 1% agarose gel containing formaldehyde on a horizontal gel electrophoresis apparatus (GIBCO BRL, Burlington, ON).

16. All parts of the gel electrophoresis apparatus, including combs, are cleaned with laboratory washing detergent and rinsed thoroughly with double-distilled water.

Notes: *It is better to use a separate set of equipment for the RNA electro-phoresis, and gloves should be worn throughout the procedure. Molecular biology grade reagents are used wherever possible.*

Reagents Needed

10 × MOPS Buffer

0.2 *M* 3-(*N*-morpholino) propane sulfonic acid (MOPS)

> 0.05 *M* sodium acetate
> 0.01 *M* EDTA (pH 7).

Loading Buffer

> 0.16 ml formaldehyde (37%)
> 0.5 ml formamide
> 10 µl 10% SDS
> 60 µl glycerol
> 4 µl 0.5 *M* EDTA
> 5 µl 1% bromophenol blue
> double-distilled water to 1 ml
> Buffer is made fresh every 2 weeks or aliquots are stored at −20°C

Running Buffer

> 18 ml formaldehyde (37%)
> 100 ml 10 × MOPS
> 882 ml double-distilled water

Ethidium bromide (10 mg/ml).

To Prepare the Agarose Gel (1%):

1. 3 g agarose, 30 ml 10 × MOPS and 255 ml water are dissolved by placing in a boiling water bath or by melting in a microwave for 2 to 3 min.
2. Allow the mixture to cool to 50°C, then add 16 µl formaldehyde (37%) and 13 µl ethidium bromide and gently mix.
3. Let the mixture cool down for about 15 min and pour the gel onto the electrophoresis plate with a comb positioned according to the manufacturer's instruction. The gel will be set in 1 to 2 hr.

To Start the Electrophoresis:

1. Calculate the volume required for 15 µg of RNA for each sample.
2. Dry the samples in a speedvac (Savant, Farmingdale, NY) for 10 to 20 min and resuspend the samples in 10 µl of DEPC-treated water.
3. Add 30 µl of loading buffer.
4. Heat the samples at 65°C for 10 min and centrifuge for 5 s to bring all the fluid down to the bottom.

5. Load samples into the wells of the agarose (1%) gel.

6. Run the gel at 30 volts overnight or until the dye migrates about 8 cm.

7. Wash the gel, using distilled water, for 30 min with gentle shaking on a platform shaker. Repeat the above process twice.

8. Photograph the gel using ultraviolet illumination with Polaroid 667 film in order to identify the 18S and 28S RNAs.

For the Northern Blot Analysis:

1. The gel is washed first with 20 × SSC for 1-2 hr (1 × SSC is 150 mM sodium chloride and 15 mM sodium citrate, pH 7.0).

2. The RNA is then transferred to Zeta-Probe GT (BioRad Laboratories) blotting membranes or nitran membranes by capillary action.

3. Place a sponge larger than the size of the gel in the bottom of a deep dish. Fill the dish half way with 20 × SSC.

4. Place three Whatman 3 mM filter paper on the sponge and soak them with 20 × SSC in water for 5 min.

5. Place the gel on top of the Whatman filter paper and remove any air bubbles by gently blotting them to the sides.

6. Cover this with Saran wrap and cut out a window so that only the gel is exposed to facilitate capillary action through the gel.

7. Place a presoaked (5 min in distilled water) Zeta-Probe membrane cut exactly to the size of the gel on top of this and carefully remove any air bubbles.

8. Soak the membrane surface with 20 × SSC buffer.

9. Place two more sheets of presoaked Whatman paper on top of the Zeta-Probe and remove any air bubbles.

10. Carefully stack paper towels on top of the Whatman paper to a height of about 15 cm.

11. Place a glass plate on top of the filters and keep pressure on the glass by using a weight (book or catalog).

Notes: *Excessive pressure can reduce the capillary transfer process. Allow the transfer to occur overnight. The transfer of RNA can be done quickly in 90 min under vacuum, using the model 785 Vacuum Blotter (BioRad Laboratories).*

12. Remove the Zeta-Probe and dry it in the air at room temperature, and then bake it at 80°C for 30 min in a vacuum oven. The RNA can also be covalently bound to the membrane by ultraviolet cross-linking with a Stratalinker (Stratagene, La Jolla, CA).

13. The dried membrane is stable at room temperature when stored dry between two filter papers and sealed in plastic bags.

The Hybridization of the RNA Immobilized on the Zeta-Probe

This proceduce is done using cDNA probes for the α and β subunits of the Na$^+$-K$^+$ ATPase. The cDNA probes are first labeled with $[\alpha^{32}P]$-dCTP by using T7 DNA polymerase and the random primer technique. The probes are separated from unincorporated radionucleotides by spinning through a Sephadex G25 column (Boehringer Mannheim, Laval, QU). About 2×10^6 cpm/ml cDNA probes are used for hybridization.

1. Seal the blotted Zeta-Probe inside a plastic bag.
2. Cut one corner of the bag and pipette in enough prehybridization buffer (50% formamide, 0.12 M Na$_2$HPO$_4$ (pH 7.2), 0.25 M NaCl, and 7% SDS) to completely soak the membrane and reseal.
3. Incubate at 43°C for 5 min.
4. Remove the solution and replace it with fresh buffer.
5. Add the probe and reseal the bag, taking care to remove all air bubbles.
6. Mix the bag thoroughly and incubate at 43°C for 4 to 24 h with thorough shaking.
7. At the end of the hybridization, remove the membrane from the bag directly into $2 \times$ SSC and wash them successively in $2 \times$ SSC, $0.5 \times$ SSS, and $0.25 \times$ SSC buffers, containing 0.1% SDS. The washing is done at room temperature for 15 min each with vigorous shaking.
8. The membranes are wrapped in plastic sheets and autoradiography is performed at –70°C with Kodak XAR-5 film using DuPont Cronex intensifying screen. The autoradiographic signals are analyzed with a BioRad Densitometer. Na$^+$-K$^+$ ATPase subunits mRNA, with respect to 18S and 28S RNA, are corrected for the difference in loading by comparing the corresponding GAPDH mRNA.

5. Summary

This article describes the techniques for the examination of Na$^+$-K$^+$ pump and associated molecular mechanisms in the intact myocardial cell. The measurements of [^{3}H]-ouabain binding and [^{86}Rb$^+$]-uptake have been given in detail, and their importance in terms of assessing the Na$^+$-K$^+$ pump activity in the myocardial cell has been emphasized. Estimation of phosphorylated intermediates, which represent the number of active Na$^+$-K$^+$ pumps, by two different techniques has been reviewed. Details concerning the measurement of Na$^+$-K$^+$

ATPase isozymes as well as mRNA abundance of Na^+-K^+ ATPase are provided to reveal the status of molecular mechanisms for changes in the enzyme activity. It is hoped that the information provided here will be helpful to the investigator in identifying functional and molecular changes in the cardiac Na^+-K^+ pump in health and disease.

Acknowledgments

The research work reported in this article was supported by a grant from the Medical Research Council of Canada (MRC Group in Experimental Cardiology).

References

1. Skou, J. C., The Na^+-K^+ pump, *News Physiol. Sci.,* 7, 95, 1992.
2. Fozzard, H. A. and Gunn, R. B., Membrane transport, in *The Heart and Cardiovascular System,* Fozzard, H. A., Jennings, B. R., Haber, E., and Katz, A. M., Eds., Raven Press, New York, 1992, chap. 6.
3. Albers, R. W., Biochemical aspects of active transport, *Annu. Rev. Biochem.,* 36, 727, 1967.
4. Post, R. L., Kume, S., Tobin, T., Orcutt, B., and Sen, A. K., Flexibility of an active centre in sodium-potassium adenosine triphosphatase, *J. Gen. Physiol.,* 54, 306S, 1969.
5. Thomas, R., Gray, P., and Andrews, J., Digitalis: its mode of action, receptor and structure-activity relationship, *Adv. Drug Res.,* 19, 311, 1990.
6. Young, R. M. and Lingrel, B.-J., Tissue distribution of mRNAs encoding the alpha isoforms and beta subunits of rat Na^+-K^+ ATPase, *Biochem. Biophys. Res. Commun.,* 145, 52, 1987.
7. Orlowski, J, and Lingrel, B.-J., Tissue specific isoform regulation of Na^+-K^+ ATPase catalytic alpha-isoforms and beta subunit mRNAs, *J. Biol. Chem.,* 263, 10436, 1988.
8. Sweadner, K. J., Isozymes of Na^+-K^+ ATPase, *Biochim. Biophys. Acta,* 988, 185, 1989.
9. Ng, Y. C. and Book, C. B., Expression of Na^+-K^+ ATPase α_1 and α_3 isoforms in adult and neonatal ferret heart, *Am. J. Physiol.,* 263, H1430, 1992.
10. Powel, T., Methods for the preparation and characterization of cardiac myocytes, in *Methods in Studying Cardiac Membrane,* vol. 1, Dhalla, N. S., Ed., CRC Press, Boca Raton, FL, 1984, chap. 4.
11. Resh, M. D., Insulin activation of (Na^+,K^+)-adenosine triphosphatase exhibits a temperature dependent lag time. Comparison to activation of the glucose transporter, *Biochemistry,* 22, 2781, 1983.

12. Hootman, S. R. and William, J. A., Sodium-potassium pump in guinea pig parotid gland: secretagogue stimulation of ouabain binding dispersed acini, *J. Physiol. (London)*, 360, 121, 1985.

13. Mandel, L. J. and Balaban, R. S., Stoichiometry and coupling of active transport to ouabain metabolism in epithelial tissue, *Am. J. Physiol.*, 240, F357, 1981.

14. Yoda, A. and Yoda, S., Interaction between ouabain and the phosphorylated intermediate of Na+,K+-ATPase, *Mol. Pharmacol.*, 22, 700, 1982.

15. Hootman, S. R. and Ernst, S. A., Estimation of Na+,K+-pump numbers and turnover in intact cells with [^{3}H] ouabain, *Methods Enzymol.*, 156, 213, 1988.

16. Mills, J. W., MacKnight, A. D. C., Jarrel, J. A., Dayer, J. M., and Ausiello, D. A., Interaction of ouabain with the Na+ pump in intact epithelial cells, *J. Cell Biol.*, 88, 637, 1981.

17. Ikenouchi, H., Zhao, L., McMillan, M., Hammond, E. M., and Barry, W. H., ATP depletion causes a reversible decrease in Na+ pump density in cultured ventricular myocytes, *Am. J. Physiol.*, 264, H1208, 1987.

18. Lobaugh, L. A. and Lieberman, M., Na+-K+ pump site density and ouabain binding affinity in cultured chick heart cells, *Am. J. Physiol.*, 253, C731, 1987.

19. Kim, D., Marsh, J. D., Barry, W. H., and Smith, T. W., Effects of growth in low potassium medium or ouabain on membrane Na+,K+-ATPase, cation transport, and contractility in cultured chick heart cells, *Circ. Res.*, 555, 39, 1984.

20. Biedert, S., Barry, W. H., and Smith, T. W., Inotropic effects and changes on sodium and calcium contents associated with inhibition of monovalent cation transport by ouabain on cultured cell, *J. Gen. Physiol. (London)*, 74, 479, 1979.

21. Lowry, O. H., Rosebrough, N. J., Farr, A. L., and Randal, R. J., Protein measurement with Folin phenol reagent, *J. Biol. Chem.*, 193, 265, 1951.

22. McPherson, G. A., Analysis of radioligand binding experiments. A collection of computer programs for the IBM-PC, *J. Pharmacol. Methods*, 14, 213, 1985.

23. Munson, P. J. and Robbard, D., Ligand: a versatile computerized approach for characterization of ligand binding systems, *Anal. Biochem.*, 107, 220, 1980.

24. English, L. H. and Schultz, J. T., Measurement of Na+-pump in isolated cells, *Methods Enzymol.*, 173, 676, 1989.

25. Akera, T., Yamamoto, S., Temmu, K., and Brody, T. M., Is ouabain-sensitive rubidium or potassium uptake a measure of sodium pump activity in isolated cardiac muscle?, *Biochim. Biophys. Acta*, 640, 779, 1981.

26. Akera, T., Methods for studying digitalis receptors, Na+-K+ ATPase and sodium pump activity in heart membrane and myocardium, in *Methods in Studying Cardiac Membrane*, Dhalla, N. S., Ed., CRC Press, Boca Raton, FL, 1984, chap. 11.

27. Albers, R. W., Koval, G. S., and Siegal, G. J., Studies on the interaction of ouabain and other cardio-active steroids with sodium-potassium activated adenosine triphosphatase, *Mol. Pharmacol.*, 4, 324, 1968.

28. Elliot, S. J. and Schilling, W. P., Oxidant stress alters Na+ pump and Na+-K+-Cl- co-transporter activities in vascular endothelial cells, *Am. J. Physiol.*, 263, H96, 1992.

29. Skou, J. C., Further investigation of a Mg^{++} + Na$^+$ activated adenosine triphosphatase, possibly related to the active linked transport of Na$^+$ and K$^+$ across the nerve membrane, *Biochim. Biophys. Acta,* 42, 6, 1960.

30. Post, R. L., Toda, G., and Rogers, F. N., Phosphorylation by inorganic phosphate of sodium plus potassium ion transport adenosine triphosphatase. Four reactive states, *J. Biol. Chem.,* 250, 69, 1975.

31. Resh, M. D., Development of insulin responsiveness of the glucose transport and the (Na$^+$,K$^+$)-adenosine triphosphatase during in vitro adipocyte differentiation, *J. Biol. Chem.,* 257, 11946, 1982.

32. Schuurman, S., Stekhorm, F. M. A. H., Swartz, H. G. P., DePont, J. J. H. H. M., and Bonting, S. L., Studies on (Na$^+$-K$^+$)-activated ATPase. XLIV. Single phosphate incorporation during dual phosphorylation by inorganic phosphate and adenosine triphosphate, *Biochim. Biophys. Acta,* 597, 100, 1980.

33. Sweadner, K. J., Two molecular forms of (Na$^+$ + K$^+$)-stimulated ATPase in brain separation and difference in affinity for strophanthidin, *J. Biol. Chem.,* 254, 6060, 1979.

34. Matsuda, T., Iwata, H., and Cooper, J. R., Specific inactivation alpha(+) molecular form of (Na$^+$ + K$^+$)-ATPase by pyrithiamin, *J. Biol. Chem.,* 259, 3858, 1984.

35. Lytton, J., Lin, J. C., and Guiodotti, G., Identification of two molecular forms of (Na$^+$ + K$^+$)-ATPase in rat adipocytes. Relation to insulin stimulation of the enzyme, *J. Biol. Chem.,* 260, 1177, 1985.

36. Laemmli, U. K., Cleavage of structural proteins during the assembly of the head of bacteriophage T$_4$, *Nature (Lond.),* 227, 680, 1970.

37. Elmosellin, A. B., Butcher, A., Samson, S. E., and Grover, A. K., Free radicals uncouple the sodium pump in pig coronary artery, *Am. J. Physiol.,* 266, C720, 1994.

38. Spencer, G. A., Yu, X., Khan, I., and Grover, A. K., Expression of isoforms of internal Ca^{2+} pump in cardiac, smooth muscle and non-muscle tissues, *Biochim. Biophys. Acta,* 1063, 15, 1991.

39. Resh, M. D., Identification and quantitation of Na$^+$-K$^+$ ATPase by back door phosphorylation, *Methods Enzymol.,* 156, 119, 1988.

40. Amory, A., Foury, F., and Goffeau, A., The purified plasma membrane ATPase of the yeast: Schizosacchromyces probe forms a phosphorylated intermediate, *J. Biol. Chem.,* 255, 9353, 1980.

41. Peterson, G. L., Ewing, R. D., Hootman, S. R., and Conte, F. P., Large scale partial purification and molecular and kinetic properties of the (Na$^+$+K$^+$)-activated adenosine triphosphatase from *Artemia salina* nauplii, *J. Biol. Chem.,* 253, 4762, 1978.

42. Sweadner, K. J., Anomalies in the electrophoretic resolution of Na$^+$/K$^+$-ATPase catalytic subunit isoforms reveal unusual protein-detergent interactions, *Biochim. Biophys. Acta,* 1029, 13, 1990.

43. Urayama, D., Shutt, H., and Sweadner, K. J., Identification of three isozymes proteins of the catalytic subunit of the Na$^+$,K$^+$ ATPase in rat brain, *J. Biol. Chem.,* 264, 8271, 1989.

44. Emanuel, J. R., Garetz, S., Stone, L., and Levenson, R., Differential expression of Na$^+$,K$^+$-ATPase α- and β-subunit mRNAs in rat tissue and cell lines, *Proc. Natl. Acad. Sci. U.S.A.,* 84, 9030, 1987.

45. McDonough, A. A., Geering, K., and Farley, R. A., The sodium pump needs its β subunit, *FASEB J.*, 4, 1605, 1990.

46. Sweadner, K. J., Multiple digitalis receptors: a molecular perspective, *Trends Cardiovasc. Med.*, 3, 2, 1993.

47. Lucchesi, P. A. and Sweadner, K. J., Postnatal changes in Na^+,K^+-ATPase isoform expression in rat cardiac ventricle: conservation of biphasic ouabain affinity, *J. Biol. Chem.*, 266, 9327, 1991.

48. Herrera, V. L., Chobamian, A. U., and Ruiz-Opazo, N., Isoform-specific modulation of Na^+,K^+-ATPase alpha-subunit gene expression in hypertension, *Science*, 241, 221, 1988.

49. Charlemagne, D., Orlowski, J., Oliviero, P., and Lane, L., mRNA accumulation of alpha and beta subunit gene of the Na^+,K^+-ATPase in hypertrophied rat heart, *J. Gen. Physiol.*, 96, 919, 1990.

50. Azuma, K. K., Hensley, C. B., Putnam, D. S., and McDonough, A. A., Hypokalemia decreases Na^+,K^+-ATPase α_2 but not α_1 isoform abundance in heart, muscle and brain, *Am. J. Physiol.*, 260, 1958, 1991.

51. Horowitz, B., Hensley, C. B., Quintero, M., Azuna, K. K., Putnam, D., and McDonough, A. A., Differential regulation of Na^+-K^+ ATPase α_1,α_2 and β subunit mRNA levels by thyroid hormone, *J. Biol. Chem.*, 265, 14308, 1990.

52. Hensley, C. B., Bershon, M. M., Sarma, J. S. M., Singh, B. N., and McDonough, A. A., Amidorone decreases Na^+,K^+-ATPase α_2 and β_2 expression specifically in cardiac ventricle, *J. Mol. Cell. Cardiol.*, 26, 417, 1994.

53. Shyjan, A. W. and Levenson, R., Antisera specific for the α_1, α_2, α_3, and β subunits of Na^+,K^+-ATPase: differential expression of α and β subunits in rat tissue membranes, *Biochemistry*, 22, 28, 1989.

54. Felsonfeld, D. P. and Sweadner, K. J., Fine specificity mapping and topography of an isozyme-specific epitope of the Na^+,K^+-ATPase catalytic subunit, *J. Biol. Chem.*, 263, 10932, 1988.

55. Burnette, W. N., "Western blotting:" electrophoretic transfer of proteins from sodium dodecyl sulfate polyacrylamide gels to unmodified nitrocellulose and radiographic detection with antibody and radioiodinated protein A, *Anal. Biochem.*, 112, 195, 1981.

56. Harris, B. A., Robishaw, J. D., Mumby, S. M., and Gilman, A. G., Molecular cloning of complementary DNA for the alpha subunit of a protein that stimulates adenylate cyclase, *Science*, 229, 1274, 1985.

57. Cox, R. A., The use of guanidinium chloride in the isolation of nucleic acids, *Methods Enzymol.*, 12 (Part B), 120, 1968.

58. Chirgwin, J. M., Przybyla, A. E., MacDonald, R. J., and Rutter, W. J., Isolation of biologically active ribonucleic acid from sources enriched in ribonuclease, *Biochemistry*, 18, 5294, 1979.

59. Chomczynski, P. and Sacchi, N., Single-step method of RNA isolation by acid guanidinium thiocyanate-phenol-chloroform extraction, *Anal. Biochem.*, 162, 156, 1987.

60. Lehrach, H. D., Diamond, D., Wozney, J. M., and Boedtker, H., RNA molecular weight determination by gel electrophoresis under denaturing condition, a critical examination, *Biochemistry*, 16, 4743, 1977.

Chapter **6**

Methods for Measuring Sodium–Hydrogen Exchange in the Heart

Hamid Massaeli and Grant N. Pierce

Contents

1. Introduction 84
2. Measurement of Sodium–Hydrogen Exchange 85
   2.1. Measurement in Sarcolemmal Membrane Vesicles 85
       2.1.1. General Approach and Precautions 85
       2.1.2. Equipment/Materials Required 86
       2.1.3. Tube Preparation and Assay Procedure 86
       2.1.4. Important Considerations 87
       2.1.5. Expected Results 89
       2.1.6. Ruling out the Involvement of Other Na^+ Transport
              Pathways 90
   2.2. Cardiomyocytes 91
       2.2.1. General Approach and Precautions 91
       2.2.2. Dye Loading Conditions and Fluorescence
              Measurement 92
       2.2.3. pH Measurement 93
       2.2.4. In Situ Calibration 96
       2.2.5. Calibration Curve Procedure 96
       2.2.6. Potential Problems 96
Acknowledgments 98
References 98

0-8493-3333-4/97/$0.00+$.50
© 1997 by CRC Press, Inc.

1. Introduction

As little as 10 years ago, the sodium–hydrogen exchange pathway attracted very little research attention from cardiovascular researchers. However, since its identification and characterization in cardiomyocytes independently by Lieberman's and Lazdunski's laboratories,[1-4] interest in the physiological and pathological roles of this pathway has increased dramatically. Further characterization of the basic biochemical properties of the exchanger in isolated cardiac sarcolemmal membranes[5,6] helped to define the possible significance of this ion transport pathway in the heart. The sodium–hydrogen exchanger appears to be a very important regulator of intracellular pH in the heart when it is in an acidic range.[4,7-9] It is either not operative or is minimally active during steady state conditions in the heart.[7,8] Lazdunski's proposal in 1985 that stimulation of the exchanger during acidic conditions in the heart such as ischemia may play an important role in reperfusion damage sparked a great deal of research on this topic.[9] Since that time, the vast majority of work directly assessing Dr. Lazdunski's hypothesis supports an important role for sodium–hydrogen exchange in ischemic–reperfusion injury (as reviewed in References 7, 10 to 12). Alterations in the sodium–hydrogen exchanger have also been demonstrated in other chronic disease states such as the diabetic cardiomyopathy.[13] This defect may impair the ability of these animals to recover from an acidic load[14] or from an ischemic challenge.[15] On the basis of our observations to date, it would be reasonable to hypothesize that the sodium–hydrogen exchanger may play a significant role in regulating intracellular pH and overall ionic homeostasis during any pathological state where a drop in intracellular pH would be expected. It is worth emphasizing that any protein which can influence intracellular pH ultimately affects the function of virtually every enzyme and process in the cell.

Three general approaches may be used to assess sodium–hydrogen exchange activity: (1) membrane biochemistry, (2) cell or tissue pharmacology, and (3) employing protein probes. Examples of the third approach would be antibody-generated immunohistochemical estimations of sodium–hydrogen exchanger density,[16] Northern blots using cDNA probes for the exchanger,[17,18] and labeled drugs that exhibit a selective affinity for the sodium–hydrogen exchanger.[19] Although these techniques provide information about exchanger density and often are used as an explanation for increases or decreases in exchange activity, they do not provide a direct measurement of exchange activity. The present treatise will not discuss these indirect measurements of activity and instead will focus on the two more direct estimations of sodium–hydrogen exchange.

2. Measurement of Sodium-Hydrogen Exchange

2.1. Measurement in Sarcolemmal Membrane Vesicles

2.1.1. General approach and precautions

The isolation of a suitable preparation of cardiac sarcolemmal vesicles will not be discussed here. The reader is referred to the appropriate methodologies[5,13,20,21] and to an excellent discussion of this topic by Dr. G.F. Tibbits (Chapter 2 in this volume). The sarcolemmal preparation must be as free as possible from contamination by other subcellular organelles and the vesicles must be intact and not "leaky." The final vesicular preparation must be taken from the sucrose gradient, washed, and suspended in a low pH solution. A typical example would be 200 mM sucrose, 25 mM MES, 8 mM KOH (pH 5.5). Be careful about the choice of buffer in which the sarcolemmal vesicles are initially suspended. If vesicles are suspended in an inappropriately buffered solution, we have found it impossible to wash out the buffer and replace it with another one efficiently enough to be useful for sodium–hydrogen exchange experiments. Vesicles can be stored in small 1- to 2-ml aliquots in plastic cryotubes, which are then snapped into metal sleeves that are in turn inserted into liquid nitrogen dewars. Vesicles can then be removed from the liquid nitrogen dewar and thawed for an experiment at the convenience of the investigator. In our hands, we have observed that the vesicular activity is unaffected by this storage procedure for up to 2 years. However, repeated freeze–thaw cycles will compromise vesicular permeability characteristics. Thus, storing the vesicles in small aliquots will help to reduce wastage when the researcher is forced to thaw the contents of a cryotube.

Sodium-hydrogen exchange can be measured in vesicles by monitoring H^+ movements or Na^+ movements. In the past, fluorescent markers sensitive to changes in pH have been used to monitor H^+ transport. Acridine orange is an example of such a dye.[22,23] However, it is used infrequently today, because it is less sensitive than radioisotopic methods. Currently, we measure sodium–hydrogen exchange as intravesicular hydrogen-dependent sodium uptake with $^{22}Na^+$ used as the marker for exchange. The principle for the assay is depicted diagrammatically in Figure 1. In the presence of a transsarcolemmal H^+ gradient, Na^+ will enter the intravesicular space. The object, therefore is to establish a suitable transsarcolemmal gradient. The interior of the vesicle is already loaded with H^+ (pH 5.5) so that a brief incubation of the vesicle with an alkaline medium will initiate the exchange of extravesicular Na^+ for intravesicular H^+. Obviously, then, any contamination of your solutions with Na^+ will produce erroneous results. The investigator must be careful to buffer the suspension medium (and any other solutions) with KOH, not NaOH. This insures that only extravesicular Na^+ is present and optimal at the start of the assay.

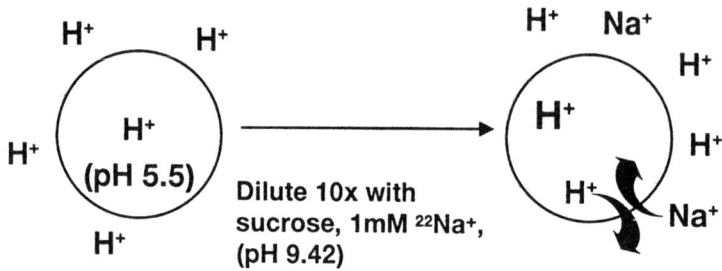

Figure 1
The principle for measuring the Na^+-H^+ exchange as intravesicular H^+-dependent $^{22}Na^+$ uptake.

2.1.2. Equipment/materials required

The equipment required for this methodology is minimal and the cost to carry out these assays would also be anticipated to be relatively small. The majority of the equipment is found in most standard biochemistry labs or, in the case of the large equipment, is frequently shared within a department.

1.   Temperature controlled water bath
2.   A set of pipettemen with adjustable volume delivery
3.   Scintillation vials (20 ml capacity)
4.   A beta scintillation counter or a gamma counter
5.   A vortex
6.   A timing device (≥ 1 s)
7.   Nitrocellulose filters (0.45 μm) Millipore
8.   Scintillation cocktail
9.   Forceps
10. Vacuum pump
11. Water bottle

2.1.3. Tube preparation and assay procedure

The steps to prepare tubes for sodium–hydrogen exchange and perform the assay are as follows:

1.   Place 5 μl of ^{22}Na (containing 0.1 μCi) on the bottom of a clear 12 $\times$ 75-mm polystyrene test tube (Symport).

2.   A 25-μl aliquot of uptake solution (200 mM sucrose, 35 mM CHES, 26 mM KOH (pH 9.42), 0.1 mM EGTA, 0.1 mM NaCl), prewarmed to 22°C, is placed with the radioisotope.

3.   A 20-μl aliquot of sarcolemmal membrane vesicles (prewarmed to 22°C) containing 20 to 30 μg of protein is placed carefully along the side of

the tube just above the uptake solution. Surface tension in the solution will keep the aliquot suspended above the uptake solution. The reaction is initiated by rapid vortexing of the mixture. The vortexing does not need to be gentle.

4. The reaction can be terminated at a preset time by the addition of 3 ml of ice-cold stop solution (100 mM KCl, 20 mM HEPES, pH 7.5) to the reaction tube followed immediately by pouring the entire volume through 0.45-μm pore size filters under vacuum. We have monitored exchange from 1 second to 2 hours.[5] Sodium–hydrogen exchange appears linear for the first 5 s of the reaction.[5] For relatively fast reaction measurements (1 to 5 s), we routinely employ an auditory signal from a timing device electronically integrated into the vortexer[24] to help us determine when to add the stop solution. For longer reaction times, careful monitoring with a simple stopwatch will provide acceptable accuracy.

5. The filters are washed twice with the vacuum still engaged with 3 ml each of the stop solution and then placed in 6 ml of a suitable scintillation fluid (e.g., Ecolume, ICN Pharmaceutical Inc., Costa Mesa, CA) for scintillation spectroscopy. The filters may also be dried and counted in a gamma counter. The results are similar.

6. Control sample tubes are required to eliminate background retention of ^{22}Na to the filters. The samples are treated in an identical way to that described above, except that the 3 ml of ice-cold stop solution is added to the assay medium prior to the addition of the vesicles. Background cpms are typically ~10% of maximal uptake, but this will vary depending upon the composition of the reaction medium.

2.1.4. Important Considerations

We will confine our discussion to specifics concerning the reaction medium and the stop solution. First, it was imperative to demonstrate that the reaction is dependent upon a transsarcolemmal H$^+$ gradient and to determine the specific characteristics of this relationship. Varying the H$^+$ concentration is easiest to perform on the extravesicular side of the membrane. However, if the investigator finds it absolutely necessary to vary the intravesicular [H$^+$], this can be done by dividing the sarcolemmal membranes into two or more groups, as they are isolated off the sucrose gradient at the end of the membrane isolation procedure, and suspending these membranes in solutions with different buffers. However, as stated, it is usually much easier to simply vary the extravesicular pH. This is not done simply by varying the pH of the uptake solution, but must be accompanied by changing the buffer to an appropriate pK for the range of pH required. For example, if the pH is required to be in the range of ~9, then CHES is an appropriate selection. Table 1 gives the pK values of a number of buffers. The pK value for the buffer is more important than the

TABLE 1
pKa Values of Selected Buffers at 25°C and 0.1 M

Buffer	Full name	pH Range	pKa
MES	2-[N-Morpholino]ethanesulfonic acid	5.5–6.7	6.1
BIS-TRIS	Bis[2-hydroxyethyl]iminotris[hydroxymethyl]-methane; 2-bis[2-hydroxyethyl]amino-2-[hydroxymethyl]-1,3-propanediol	5.8–7.2	6.5
ADA	N-[2-Acetamido]-2-iminodiacetic acid; N-[carbamoylmethyl] iminodiacetic acid	6.0–7.2	6.6
ACES	2-[(2-Amino-2-oxoethyl)amino]ethanesulfonic acid; N-[2acetamido]-2-aminoethane-sulfonic acid	6.1–7.5	6.8
PIPES	Piperazine–N,N'-bis[2-ethanesulfonic acid]; 1,4-piperazinediethane sulfonic acid	6.1–7.5	6.8
MOPSO BIS-TRIS	3-[N-Morpholino]-2-hydroxypropanesulfonic acid	6.2–7.6	6.9
PROPANE	1,3-Bis[tris(hydroxymethyl-O-methylamino]propane	6.3–9.5	6.8, 9.0
BES	N,N-Bis[2-hydroxyethyl]-2-aminoethanesulfonic acid; 2-[bis(2-hydroxyethyl)amino] ethanesulfonic acid	6.4–7.8	7.1
MOPS	3-[N-Morpholino]propanesulfonic acid	6.5–7.9	7.2
TES	N-Tris[hydroxymethyl]methyl-2-aminoethanesulfonic acid; 2-([2-hydroxy 1,1-bis (hydroxymethyl)ethyl]amino)ethanesulfonic acid	6.8–8.2	7.4
HEPES	N-[2-Hydroxyethyl]piperazine-N'-[2-ethanesulfonic acid]	6.8–8.2	7.5
DIPSO	3-[N,N-Bis(2-hydroxyethyl)amino]-2-hydroxy-propanesulfonic acid	7.0–8.2	7.6
TAPSO	3-[N-Tris(hydroxymethyl)methylamino]-2-hydroxypropanesulfonic acid	7.0–8.2	7.6
TRIZMA	Tris[hydroxymethyl]aminomethane	7.0–9.2	8.1
HEPPSO	N-[2-Hydroxyethyl]piperazine-N'-[2-hydroxypropanesulfonic acid]	7.1–8.5	7.8
POPSO	Piperazine-N,N'-bis[2-hydroxypropanesulfonic acid]	7.2–8.5	7.8
EPPS	N-[2-Hydroxyethyl]piperazine-N'-[3-propanesulfonic acid]; HEPPS	7.3–8.7	8.0
TEA	Triethanolamine (2,2',2''-Nitrilotriethanol)	7.3–8.3	7.8
TRICINE	N-Tris[hydroxymethyl]methylglycine; N-[2-hydroxy-1,1-bis (hydroxymethyl) ethyl] glycine	7.4–8.8	8.1
BICINE	N,N-Bis[2-hydroxyethyl]glycine	7.6–9.0	8.3
TAPS	N-Tris[hydroxymethyl]methyl-3-aminopropanesulfonic acid; ([2-hydroxy-1,1-bis (hydroxymethyl)-ethyl]amino)-1-propanesulfonic acid	7.7–9.1	8.4
AMPSO	3-[(1,1-Dimethyl-2-hydroxyethyl)amino]-2-hydroxypropanesulfonic acid	8.3–9.7	9.0
CHES	2-[N[Cyclohexylamino]ethanesulfonic acid	8.6–10.0	9.3

TABLE 1 (continued)
pKa Values of Selected Buffers at 25°C and 0.1 M

Buffer	Full name	pH Range	pKa
CAPSO	3-[Cyclohexylamino]-2-hydroxy-1-propanesulfonic acid	8.9–10.3	9.6
AMP	2-Amino-2-methyl-1-propanol	9.0–10.5	9.7
CAPS	3-[Cyclohexylamino]-1-propanesulfonic acid	9.7–11.1	10.4

buffer range. These are not the only buffers which could be used, but represent a list of conventional buffers.

The final extravesicular pH of the reaction medium is actually a combination of the interaction of 20 µl of sarcolemmal vesicles at pH 5.5 and 25 µl of uptake solution at, for example, pH 10.61.[5] The final extravesicular pH was determined by direct measurement with a pH electrode to be 9.33. We determined the final pH of all of the media empirically in preliminary experiments whenever sodium–hydrogen exchange was to be measured as a function of the [H⁺] of the extravesicular solution.[5]

Second, the composition of the stop solution is important. Different ions can influence sodium–hydrogen exchange.[23,25] It is possible, then, that the stop solution may interact with the transsarcolemmal Na^+ movements instead of simply stopping them. However, we have found that KCl was necessary in the stop solution to reduce background counts (probably by removing ^{22}Na from the extravesicular membrane binding sites and from nonspecific binding to the filters). The addition of amiloride, a known blocker of sodium–hydrogen exchange,[5] to the stop solution was without effect. The 9 ml volume for stopping and washing the filters was found to be the optimal amount required to reduce background counts.

2.1.5. Expected Results

Typical results depicting intravesicular H^+-dependent Na^+ uptake as a function of reaction time are shown in Figure 2. Drugs like amiloride which are known inhibitors of sodium–hydrogen exchange, block sarcolemmal Na^+ uptake in our assay system in an expected manner.[5,13] The values shown here for rat cardiac sarcolemmal vesicles are similar to activities exhibited previously for canine[5] and bovine[23] cardiac sarcolemma.

The results shown in Figure 2 are calculated as follows. The cpm values at the 10 s time point, for example, were 1075 and 99 for the uptake and blank tubes, respectively. The tube contained 41.32 µg sarcolemmal protein. A 50-µl aliquot of the ^{22}Na stock produced 156,521 cpm. The Na^+ concentration of the assay was 0.05 mM. The calculations were made according to the equation:

$$\frac{\text{ml standard}}{\text{cpm standard}} \times \frac{\text{nmol } Na^+/\text{ml}}{\text{mg protein}} \times \Delta \text{ sample cpm} = \text{nmole } Na^+/\text{mg protein}$$

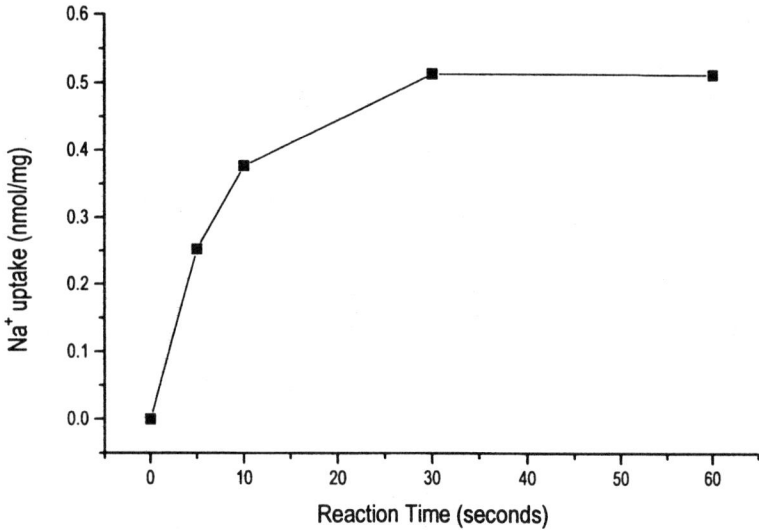

Figure 2
Results from a representative experiment showing Na⁺ uptake via Na⁺-H⁺ exchange in rat cardiac
sarcolemmal vesicles as a function of reaction time.

Thus, in the above experiment we had:

$$\frac{0.05}{156,521} \times \frac{50}{0.04132} \times (1075 - 99) = 0.377 \text{ nmole Na}^+/\text{mg protein}$$

2.1.6. Ruling out the involvement of other Na⁺ transport pathways

It is always possible that Na⁺ transport pathways other than sodium–hydrogen
exchange may contribute to the ²²Na movements that we are measuring. However, one of the strengths of the vesicular biochemical work is the ability to
precisely manipulate the reaction environment and accurately isolate the
sodium–hydrogen exchanger. Several potential Na⁺ transport pathways must
be considered. The Na⁺ pump is unlikely to contribute to the ²²Na uptake
measured in our assay because this pump requires energy and ATP is not
present in the reaction media. The uptake of ²²Na is also insensitive to blockers
of the Na⁺ pump like ouabain. Voltage sensitive Na⁺ channel participation is
also unlikely, because exchange is not influenced by interventions which would
alter transsarcolemmal charge distribution.[6,25] The participation of Na⁺/Ca²⁺
exchange in the reaction is also unlikely for several reasons. First, Li⁺ is a
relatively poor inhibitor of Na⁺/Ca²⁺ exchange,[26] yet it is a potent inhibitor of
²²Na uptake under our assay conditions.[5] Second, the presence of EGTA in
the reaction media should have chelated all of the Ca²⁺ available to participate

in such a reaction.[5] Finally, the Na^+/Ca^{2+} exchanger and all of the other Na^+ transport processes identified (Na^+ pump, Na^+ channels) would be inhibited by an intravesicular pH of 5.5. Thus, it is reasonable to conclude that we are biochemically dissecting out an accurate measurement of sodium–hydrogen exchange.

2.2.   Cardiomyocytes

2.2.1.   General approach and precautions

There are advantages and limitations to consider when one measures sodium–hydrogen exchange in cardiomyocytes. The primary advantage of using a single cardiomyocyte as the model of investigation is that it provides a closer representation of *in vivo* conditions. The ionic milieu is more physiological than those used in biochemical studies and the cells are presumably less altered during the isolation procedure than are sarcolemmal membrane preparations. The disadvantages include the potential problems that other transport pathways may induce on ion flux through the exchanger and the possibility that intracellular compartmentation of Na^+ or H^+ may influence the activity of the exchanger. Complications in dye dynamics (if a dye is used to monitor the ion movements) will also add to the complexity of the measurement. However, the ability to measure sodium–hydrogen exchange simultaneously with other ion movements[27] and other aspects of cell function (i.e., contractility) is an overwhelming benefit which can be invaluable in both physiological and pathological studies.

Sodium–hydrogen exchange can be monitored in cells by following ^{22}Na movements[28] or monitoring fluorescent dyes sensitive to H^+ or Na^+. The former technique is less than optimal because: (1) the measurement is not on-line and continuous; (2) there are serious limitations introduced by washing a cell prior to measuring its ion content; (3) the cell is destroyed during the measurement process; and (4) because of (3), the same cell cannot be used as its own control. These limitations can introduce important errors in ion flux measurement and conclusions.[29]

Molecules that have absorbed light exist in a higher electronic state and must lose this excess energy to return to their basal charge. A molecule which returns to its basal state by emitting light demonstrates photoluminescence. Luminescence, or fluorescence, therefore, is a phenomenon where previously absorbed light is re-emitted from a molecule. Fluorescence is usually found in molecules that are aromatic or which contain multiple-conjugated double bonds with great resonance stability. Compounds useful in cell biological applications have been designed which possess two important features. First, they are highly fluorescent, and second, they are relatively specific for a stimulation of this fluorescence. Fluorescent spectroscopy is one of the most sensitive, least disruptive methodologies available to monitor ionic homeostasis in cells. It permits relatively fast resolution of ionic movements over a continuous period of time. More than one ion can be monitored simultaneously in the same cell loaded with different dyes.[27] Intracellular and even intercellular ion movements can be monitored with conventional fluorescent spectrofluorometers, or additional data can be obtained with a UV-confocal microscope.[30] The equipment needed is relatively expensive and accessible to only one investigator at a time. However, the power of this technique has outweighed any potential disadvantages and fluorescent microscopy is now a widely used and accepted biological technique.

The isolation of a suitable preparation of cardiomyocytes is essential for the success of this technique. Appropriate methodology for the isolation of cardiomyocytes is described in detail in Chapter 7 of this volume (by Rodrigues and Severson). Although many other dyes are available, two dyes are most commonly used to monitor intracellular pH: BCECF ($2',7'$ bis(carboxyethyl)-5(6)-carboxyfluorescein) or SNARF-1. BCECF is a dual-excitation, single-emission dye, whereas SNARF-1 is a single-excitation, dual emission probe. Choosing to use one or the other will largely depend upon the physical characteristics of your spectrofluorometer system. Both dyes can be loaded into the cells, either in the acid form or in the esterified form. The dyes can be loaded passively or via microinjection through pipettes. The protocols for loading cells with these dyes is similar for both BCECF and SNARF. We will describe the methodology using BCECF, but the general technique is applicable to SNARF as well.

2.2.2.   Dye loading conditions and fluorescence measurement

BCECF-AM (acetoxymethyl ester of BCECF) was obtained from Molecular Probes in special packaging (50 µg per vial). This is important if a small quantity of BCECF is to be used as a stock solution each time. A 1-mM stock solution of BCECF-AM was prepared in dry DMSO and kept frozen at $-20°C$ until use. The ester form of BCECF is a nonfluorescent molecule, and it will fluoresce upon de-esterification. Therefore, any highly colored BCECF-AM stock solution should be discarded.

Cardiomyocytes can be loaded with BCECF, either in suspension or in cells already attached to coverslips. These cells were incubated in a physiological solution (i.e., (in mM) 135 NaCl, 5 KCl, 1.8 CaCl$_2$, 1 MgCl$_2$, 8 dextrose, 10 HEPES) with 2 µM BCECF-AM for approximately 20 min at 23°C. The loading conditions may vary from investigator to investigator. However, it is important to complete preliminary tests to determine the optimal conditions.

BCECF-AM is a lipophilic molecule and enters the cell easily. Once within the cell, the acetoxymethyl ester will be cleaved by the action of cytoplasmic esterases. This will result in entrapment of BCECF within the cytoplasm. The loaded cells are then washed with a physiological solution 3 times to remove any extracellular BCECF (esterified and unesterified).

2.2.3. pH Measurement

The following sections will describe in detail the procedures necessary to measure intracellular pH in single cells with a fluorescent indicator dye. Once appropriate signals are obtained, these can be converted into units of [H⁺] through calibration techniques if necessary. However, this is not always mandatory if one is simply interested in qualitative data. BCECF is a dual-excitation, single emission dye. It can be excited at the absorption maximum 500 to 505 nm and the isosbestic point (wavelength at which the emission intensity does not change with different concentrations of hydrogen ion) 440 nm, and its emission can be recorded in the 525 to 530 nm range. BCECF has a pKa of 6.97. Therefore, its fluorescence ratio is linear between pH 6 and 8 (Figure 3). This property of BCECF makes it ideal for measuring pH in the physiological range.

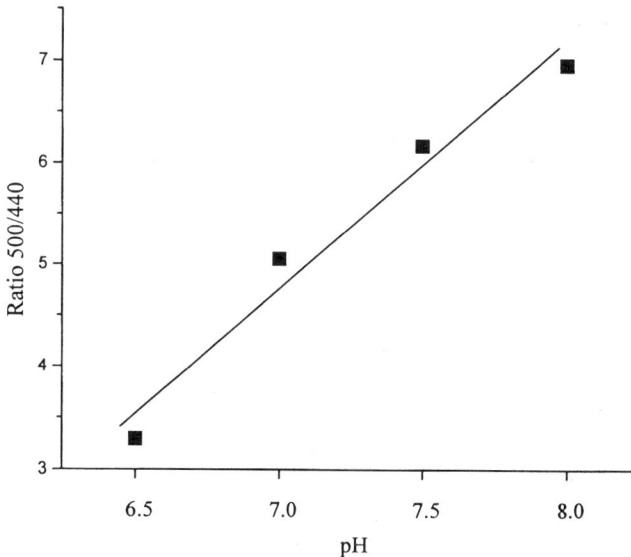

Figure 3

In situ calibration curve of BCECF-loaded cardiomyocytes. This fluorescence ratio was obtained (by exciting the cardiomyocytes at 440 and 500 nm and recording emission at 525 nm) with different pH standard solutions containing high K⁺ and nigericin. The fluorescence ratio is linear between pH 6.5 and 8.0 (R = 0.984).

To begin measurement of intracellular pH

1. Turn on the xenon lamp connected to a SPEX Fluorolog spectrofluorometer (SPEX Industries, Edison, NJ) (Figure 4) or a similar instrument. In order to prevent any damage to the computer and other electronic devices from power surge, it is very important to turn on the lamp first. The SPEX system is connected to a Nikon Diaphot epifluorescent

microscope with a set of 100×, 40× oil CF Epi-Fluorescence Fluor, and 20× PL2 objectives (available to us).

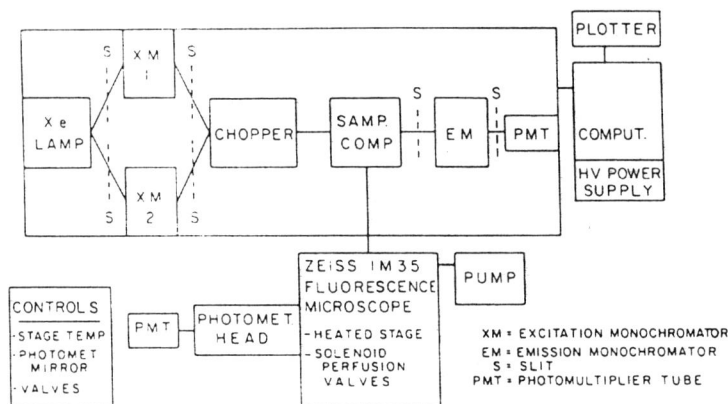

Figure 4
Schematic of the SPEX Fluorolog spectrofluorometer system currently in use in our laboratory. It can be integrated with a Nikon Diaphot, a Zeiss IM35, or any other suitable fluorescent microscope for visualization of the cells.

2. Turn down the lights in the laboratory. It is a good idea to cover the microscope with a dark curtain to prevent stray light from entering into the optical path.

3. Set the excitation wavelength by adjusting the monochromators to 440 and 500 nm and the emission wavelength to 525. Use a filter block with the proper dichroic mirror and barrier filters. We used a Nikon DM510 filter block, because it contains a 510 nm dichroic mirror and a 520 nm barrier filter.

4. Place the coverslip with the BCECF-loaded cardiomyocytes in the coverslip holding device (Leiden coverslip dish, Medical System Corp., Greenval, NY), and add 1 ml of physiological solution (as described above).

5. Turn on the temperature regulator and set it to the desired temperature (37°C).

6. Use the stage control on the microscope to find the desired cardiomyocyte (i.e., cylindrical in shape and responding to electrical stimulation) and center the cell in the measurement field.

7. Start collecting data from a single cell. At this stage you should be able to see two traces, one for 440 nm and a second one for 500 nm (but with higher intensity). These traces represent the basal pH level. Furthermore, the ratio of 500/440 represents the change in pH.

A simple technique to measure intracellular pH regulation

Na^+-H^+ exchange plays an important role in regulating intracellular pH. The simplest way to study this regulation is to load the cardiomyocytes with acid and observe the recovery, as follows:

1. Load the cardiomyocytes and prepare them for pH measurement as described above.

2. Start recording resting intracellular pH from a single cell.

3. Add 20 mM NH$_4$Cl (final concentration) to the cardiomyocytes (Figure 5). Addition of NH$_4$Cl will result in a rapid increase in intracellular pH due to the entry of NH$_3$. This increase will plateau due to a slower entry of NH$^+_4$ and protonation of the NH$_3$ to generate more NH$^+_4$. After washing out the extracellular NH$_4$Cl, the intracellular NH$_3$ will passively move out of the cardiomyocytes, down its concentration gradient, leaving behind the H$^+$. This build-up of H$^+$ in the cytoplasm will further activate the Na$^+$-H$^+$ exchanger. The exchanger activity will remove excess H$^+$ to neutralize the intracellular pH. It is very important to use a bicarbonate-free solution, in order to isolate the Na$^+$-H$^+$ exchanger activity. The presence of bicarbonate in the extracellular space will activate other pH$_i$ regulating systems (i.e., the anion exchanger Cl$^-$/HCO$_3^-$ or Na$^+$/HCO$_3^-$ co-transport).[34,35]

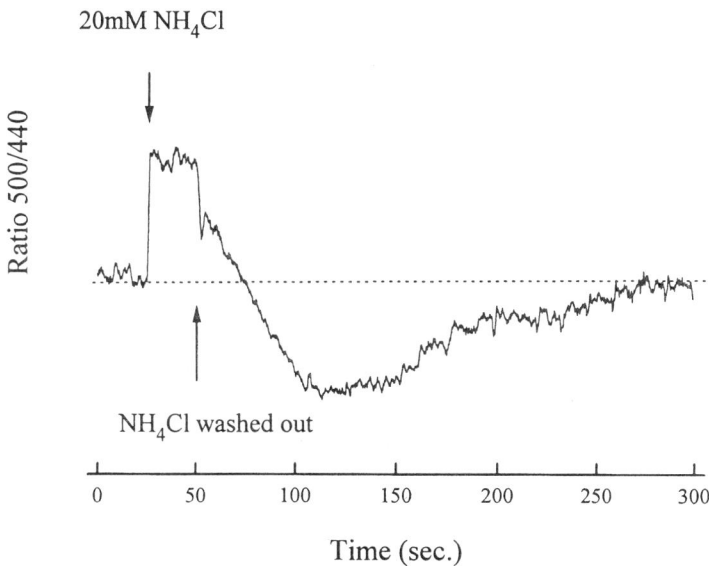

Figure 5

Role of Na$^+$/H$^+$ exchanger in regulating pH$_i$ after acid load. NH$_4$Cl (20 mM) was added to the cardiomyocytes and then removed (as shown by arrows).

2.2.4. In situ calibration

Calibration of the BCECF fluorescence ratio is carried out by using nigericin (H^+/K^+ ionophore). Nigericin equilibrates the intracellular and extracellular $[H^+]$ to the intracellular and extracellular $[K^+]$ (i.e., $[K^+]_i/[K^+]_o = [H^+]_i/[H^+]_o$). Therefore, by equilibrating the $[K^+]_o$ to the $[K^+]_i$ in the presence of nigericin, then the $[H^+]_i$ will be equal to the $[H^+]_o$.[32] However, it is important to remove all Na^+ from the extracellular space, by washing the cells with high KCl solution.

2.2.5. Calibration curve procedure

1. Prepare a physiological solution containing high KCl (i.e., (in mM): 0 NaCl, 140 KCl, 1 CaCl$_2$, 1 MgCl$_2$, 8 dextrose, 10 HEPES, and without bicarbonate). Use this solution to make 5 or more pH standard solutions (i.e., pH 6.5, 7, 7.5, 8). For this step it is important to use an accurate pH meter.

2. Add 7 μM nigericin (Sigma Canada, Ltd.) dissolved in ethanol to each of these standards.

3. Place the coverslip with BCECF-loaded cardiomyocytes in the Leiden dish, and add 1 ml high K^+/nigericin solution pH 7.4.

4. Start recording for 50 s at pH 7.4. This time can be changed as desired.

5. Superfuse the cell (with a low flow pump and an appropriate aspirator to remove the fluid) for a couple of minutes with the pH 6.5 standard solution, or gently wash the cells 3 to 4 times with the pH 6.5 standard solution. The temperature of the standards should be adjusted to 37°C.

6. Once the cardiomyocytes are equilibrated in the new standard solution, allow some time for a steady state to be attained.

7. Start recording again for another 50 s.

8. Repeat steps 5 to 7 for each pH standard solution.

9. Typically, the fluorescence intensity at 440 nm (isosbestic point) should not change with different pHs, but the intensity at 500 nm is dependent upon the intracellular pH (see Figure 6).

10. For an accurate quantification of pH$_i$, it is important to do this calibration curve after each experiment. However, there is another way to convert the fluorescence ratio to pH$_i$ by using a similar formula as used for $[Ca^{2+}]_i$ measurements with fura-2 (for details see James-Kracke[33]).

2.2.6. Potential problems

One of the major problems with using BCECF is the extent of dye loading into the cell. BCECF loading depends on several factors such as the cell type, membrane integrity of the isolated cells, temperature, time, dye concentration, and esterase activity. Any of the above factors may cause poor loading and a weak fluorescent signal. In our hands, a weak signal is anything recorded by

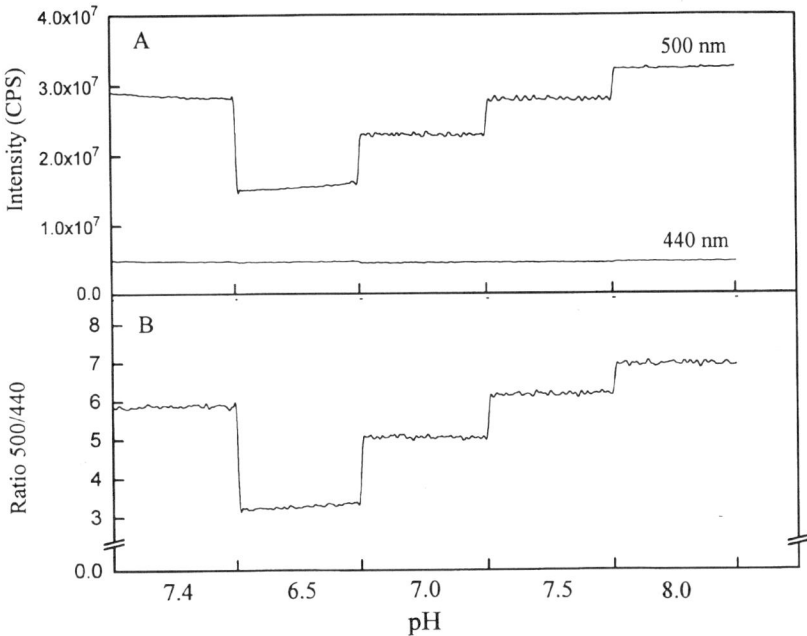

Figure 6

In situ calibration of BCECF fluorescent. Panel **A**: excitation intensities at 440 nm (isosbestic point) and 500 nm after exposure of cell to solutions with a different pH. Panel **B**: BCECF fluorescence ratio of 500/440. (From Pierce, G.N. et al., *J. Pharmacol. Exp. Ther.*, 265, 1280, 1993. With permission.)

the photomultiplier tube which is in the intensity range of 1×10^5 counts per second or below. Factors such as the temperature, time, and dye concentration could be manipulated to obtain the optimum condition for different cells. Using esterified probes for cell loading could generate further problems such as compartmentation of the dye, uneven loading within the same population of cells, extracellular deesterification of the dye (mostly in the presence of serum). However, in cardiomyocytes, only 8% of BCECF fluorescence was compartmentalized in intracellular organelles.[31] The extent of compartmentation can be tested by treating cardiomyocytes with digitonin. This will result in removal of the cytoplasmic BCECF, while the trapped BCECF remains in the cell. However, compartmentation could be minimized by microinjecting the acid form of BCECF into the cells.

Another important factor that will affect the fluorescence intensity is photobleaching. The extent of photobleaching can be determined by measuring the fluorescence intensity at 440 nm (isosbestic point) for a period of time. At this isosbestic point, the intensity of fluorescence is not affected by change in pH_i. Therefore, any decrease in fluorescence intensity over a period of time corresponds to photobleaching. It is possible to decrease the photobleaching by reducing either the excitation light intensity or time of exposure.

Of course, it is critical before the researcher undertakes any study of ion movements via fluorescent techniques that the functional viability of the cell under investigation be insured. In cardiomyocytes, measurement of the resting electrical membrane potential (~ -80 mV), cell shape (elongated, cylindrical), a lack of spontaneous contractile activity at rest, and contractile response after electrical stimulation are all good tests of cell integrity. If the dye does not work in cells after these criteria have been met, it is likely that the problem does not reside with the cells. Oxygenation of the cells during experiments is mandatory if the cells are to remain viable for many hours (up to ~5 hours after the isolation and dye loading is complete). Cells can be used immediately after completion of the collagenase isolation procedure once it has been ascertained that the cells are viable and Ca^{2+} tolerant.

Acknowledgments

This work was supported by the Heart and Stroke Foundation of Manitoba. Hamid Massaeli was a trainee of the Heart and Stroke Foundation of Canada. Grant N. Pierce was a Scientist of the Medical Research Council of Canada.

References

1. Piwnica-Worms, D. and Lieberman, M., Microfluorometric monitoring of pH_i in cultured heart cells: Na^+-H^+ exchange, *Am. J. Physiol.*, 244, C422, 1983.
2. Piwnica-Worms, D., Jacob, R., Horres, C.R., and Lieberman, M., Na^+/H^+ exchange in cultured chick heart cells, *J. Gen. Physiol.*, 85, 43, 1985.
3. Frelin, C., Vigne, P., and Lazdunski, M., The role of the Na^+/H^+ exchange system in cardiac cells in relation to the control of the internal Na^+ concentration, *J. Biol. Chem.*, 259, 8880, 1984.
4. Frelin, C., Vigne, P., and Lazdunski, M., The role of the Na^+/H^+ exchange system in the regulation of the internal pH in cultured cardiac cells, *Eur. J. Biochem.*, 149, 1, 1985.
5. Pierce, G.N. and Philipson, K.D., Na^+/H^+ exchange in cardiac sarcolemmal vesicles, *Biochim. Biophys. Acta*, 818, 109, 1985.
6. Seiler, S.M., Cragoe, E.J., and Jones, L.R., Demonstration of a Na^+/H^+ exchange activity in purified canine cardiac sarcolemmal vesicles, *J. Biol. Chem.*, 260, 4869, 1985.
7. Fliegel, L. and Frohlich, O., The Na^+/H^+ exchanger: an update on structure, regulation and cardiac physiology, *Biochem. J.*, 296, 273, 1993.
8. Pierce, G.N., Cole, W.C., Liu, K., Massaeli, H., Maddaford, T.G., Chen, Y.J., et al., Modulation of cardiac performance by amiloride and several selected derivatives of amiloride, *J. Pharmacol. Exp. Ther.*, 265, 1280, 1993.

9. Lazdunski, M., Frelin, C., and Vigne, P., The sodium/hydrogen exchange system in cardiac cells: its biochemical and pharmacological properties and its role in regulating internal concentrations of sodium and internal pH, *J. Mol. Cell Cardiol.*, 17, 1029, 1985.

10. Pierce, G.N. and Czubryt, M.P., The contribution of ionic imbalance to ischemia/reperfusion-induced injury, *J. Mol. Cell. Cardiol.*, 27, 53, 1995.

11. Pierce, G.N. and Meng, H., The role of sodium-proton exchange in ischemic/reperfusion injury in the heart, *Am. J. Cardiovasc. Pathol.*, 4, 91, 1992.

12. Karmazyn, M., Ischemic and reperfusion injury in the heart. Cellular mechanisms and pharmacological interventions, *Can. J. Physiol. Pharmacol.*, 69, 719, 1991.

13. Pierce, G.N., Ramjiawan, B., Dhalla, N.S., and Ferrari, R., Na^+/H^+ exchange in cardiac sarcolemmal vesicles isolated from diabetic rats, *Am. J. Physiol.*, 258, H255, 1990.

14. Lagadic-Gossman, D., Chesnais, J.M., and Feuvray, D., Intracellular pH regulation in papillary muscle cells from streptozotocin diabetic rats: an ion-sensitive microelectrode study, *Pflügers Arch.*, 412, 613, 1988.

15. Tani, M. and Neely, J.R., Hearts from diabetic rats are more resistant to in vitro ischemia: possible role of altered Ca^{2+} metabolism, *Circ. Res.*, 62, 931, 1988.

16. Kleyman, T.R. and Zebrowitz, J.R., Distinct epitopes on amiloride. II. Variably restricted epitopes defined by monoclonal anti-amiloride antibodies, *Am. J. Physiol.*, 260, C271, 1991.

17. Dyck, J.R.B., Maddaford, T.G., Pierce, G.N., and Fliegel, L., Induction of expression of the Na^+/H^+ exchanger in the rat myocardium, *Cardiovasc. Res.*, 29, 203, 1995.

18. Dyck, J.R.B., Lopaschuk, G.D., and Fliegel, L., Identification of a small Na^+/H^+ exchanger-like message in the rabbit myocardium, *FEBS Lett.*, 310, 255, 1992.

19. Ross, W., Bertrand, W., and Morrison, A., A photoactivatable probe for the Na^+/H^+ exchanger cross-links a 66-kDa renal brush border membrane protein, *J. Biol. Chem.*, 265, 5341, 1990.

20. Kutryk, M.J.B. and Pierce, G.N., Stimulation of sodium-calcium exchange by cholesterol incorporation into isolated cardiac sarcolemmal vesicles, *J. Biol. Chem.*, 263, 13167, 1988.

21. Dhalla, N.S. and Pierce, G.N., *Methods In Studying Cardiac Membranes*, vol. 1, CRC Press, Boca Raton, FL, 1984, 3.

22. Ives, H.E., Yee, V.J., and Warnock, D.G., Mixed type inhibition of the renal Na^+/H^+ antiporter by Li^+ and amiloride, *J. Biol. Chem.*, 258, 9710, 1983.

23. Periyasamy, S.M., Kakar, S.S., Garlid, K.D., and Askari, A., Ion specificity of cardiac sarcolemmal Na^+/H^+ antiporter, *J. Biol. Chem.*, 265, 6035, 1990.

24. Philipson, K.D., *Methods in Studying Cardiac Membranes*, vol. 1, CRC Press, Boca Raton, FL, 1984, 147.

25. Pierce, G.N., Cationic interactions with Na^+/H^+ exchange and passive Na^+ flux in cardiac sarcolemmal vesicles, *Mol. Cell. Biochem.*, 78, 89, 1987.

26. Philipson, K.D. and Nishimoto, A.Y., Efflux of Ca^{2+} from cardiac sarcolemmal vesicles, Influence of external Ca^{2+} and Na^+, *J. Biol. Chem.*, 256, 3698, 1981.

27. Martinez-Zaguilan, R., Martinez, G.M., Lattanzio, F., and Gillies, R.J., Simultaneous measurement of intracellular pH and Ca^{2+} using the fluorescence of SNARF-1 and fura-2, *Am. J. Physiol.*, 260, C297, 1991.

28. Soleimani, M., Bookstein, C., McAteer, J.A., Hattabaugh, Y.J., Bizal, G.L., Musch, M.W. et al., Effect of high osmolality on Na^+/H^+ exchange in renal proximal tubule cells, *J. Biol. Chem.*, 269, 15613, 1994.

29. Pierce, G.N., Langer, G.A., Wright, G.B., and Kutryk, M.J.B., Calcium is rapidly exchangeable in cultured vascular smooth muscle cells from rabbit aorta, *J. Mol. Cell. Cardiol.*, 21, 889, 1989.

30. Chacon, E., Reece, J.M., Neiminen, A.L., Zahreblski, G., Herman, B., and Lemasters, J.J., Distribution of electrical potential, pH, free Ca^{2+}, and volume inside cultured adult rabbit cardiac myocytes during hypoxia: a multiparameter digitized confocal microscopy study, *Biophys. J.*, 66, 942, 1994.

31. Borzak, S., Kelly, R.A., Krämer, B.K., Matoba, Y., Marsh, J.D., and Reers, M., *In situ* calibration of fura-2 and BCECF fluorescence in adult rat ventricular myocytes, *Am. J. Physiol.*, 259, H973, 1990.

32. Weissberg, P.L., Little, P.J., Cargoe, E.J., Jr., and Bobik, A., Na-H antiport in cultured rat aortic smooth muscle: its role in cytoplasmic pH regulation, *Am. J. Physiol.*, 253, C193, 1987.

33. James-Kracke, M.R., Quick and accurate method to convert BCECF fluorescence to pH_i: calibration in three different type of cell preparations, *J. Cell Physiol.*, 151, 596, 1992.

34. Reinertsen, K.V., Tønnessen, T.I., Jacobsen, J., Sandvig, K., and Olses, S., Role of chloride/bicarbonate antiport in the control of cytosolic pH, *J. Biol. Chem.*, 263, 11117, 1988.

35. Cassel, D., Scharf, O., Rotman, M., Cragoe, E.J., Jr., and Katz, M., Characterization of Na^+-linked and Na^+-independent Cl^-/HCO_3^- exchange systems in Chinese hamster lung fibroblasts, *J. Biol. Chem.*, 263, 6122, 1988.

Chapter

Preparation of Cardiomyocytes

Brian Rodrigues and David L. Severson

Contents

1. Introduction 102
   1.1. Uses of Isolated Cardiomyocytes 102
        1.1.1. Electrophysiology 102
        1.1.2. Metabolism 102
        1.1.3. Contractility 103
        1.1.4. Assay of Enzymes and Isolation of Intracellular
               Organelles 103
        1.1.5. Receptors and Signal Transduction Mechanisms 104
        1.1.6. Pathophysiological Studies 104
   1.2. Limitations 104
   1.3. History of Isolation Procedures 104
2. Methodology for Isolating Cardiomyocytes 105
   2.1. Preparation of Solutions 106
   2.2. Heart Perfusion 107
   2.3. Isolation of Cardiomyocytes 108
   2.4. Determination of Yield and Viability 109
   2.5. Potential Problems 111
        2.5.1. Poor Dissociation of Hearts 112
        2.5.2. Low Viability of Isolated Cardiomyocytes 112
Acknowledgments 113
References 113

0-8493-3333-4/97/$0.00+$.50
© 1997 by CRC Press, Inc.

101

1. Introduction

The cellular heterogeneity of the heart can be a complicating factor in experimental studies of cardiac function. Although cardiomyocytes comprise the majority (80%) of the heart's mass, myocytes make up only about 25% of the total number of cardiac cells.[1] Smooth muscle and endothelial cells from the coronary vasculature, fibroblasts, neural elements, and even adipocytes are all present in the whole heart. Microscopic studies coupled with *in situ* hybridization and immunocytochemistry can provide specific information concerning mRNA and protein expression in specific cell types in the heart,[2,3] but these techniques have only a restricted application to studies of cardiac function. The availability of procedures to isolate cardiomyocytes offers an extremely useful experimental tool; studies can be conducted with a homogeneous cell population where the extracellular environment can be carefully controlled and manipulated.[4] Cardiomyocytes have been isolated successfully from the hearts of many species,[5] but rat hearts are used most commonly. The experimental advantages associated with the use of isolated cardiomyocytes to study cardiac function are illustrated in the following examples.

1.1. Uses of Isolated Cardiomyocytes

1.1.1. Electrophysiology

Isolated cardiomyocytes retain the electrophysiological characteristics of intact muscle preparations with respect to resting membrane potential and action potential configuration.[4] Specific ion currents (e.g., L-type Ca^{2+} channels) can be measured by voltage clamping in the whole cell mode. Multicellular cardiac preparations with a functional syncytium are much less suitable for voltage clamping.[5] Isolated cardiomyocytes can also be utilized effectively for patch-clamp studies to identify specific ion channels. Since electrophysiological recordings are measured using single cells impaled by a microelectrode, these studies can be conducted with a small number of cells isolated from specific regions of the heart such as pacemaker tissues (e.g., SA node)[6] or even epicardial and endocardial cells from ventricular tissue.[7]

1.1.2. Metabolism

Isolated cardiomyocytes can be incubated under defined conditions so that the time dependence and regulation of various metabolic processes can be studied. Bihler et al.[8] utilized cardiomyocytes to study the calcium dependence of glucose transport; variations in cell isolation procedures and incubation conditions produced marked changes in glucose uptake. Cardiomyocytes also provide the opportunity to show that specific metabolic pathways are present in myocytes. For example, Kryski et al.[9] showed that isoproterenol- stimulated lipolysis (mobilization of endogenous triacylglycerols) occurred in cardiomyocytes. Previously, lipolysis had only been studied in whole perfused hearts where the contribution of other cell types (e.g., cardio-adipocytes) to this metabolic pathway could not be excluded. Also, isolated ventricular cardiomyocytes are quiescent because the resting membrane potential is stable, except for a few slow wave contractions due to spontaneous Ca^{2+} release from the sarcoplasmic reticulum (SR).[5] Therefore, the direct metabolic effects of agents such as beta-adrenergic agonists can be studied with cardiomyocytes, because the confounding influence of an increased ATP demand that is produced by the inotropic response in a whole perfused heart which can secondarily influence myocardial metabolism is eliminated.

1.1.3.   Contractility

Quiescent cardiomyocytes will contract in response to electrical field stimulation; mechanical or optical detection is used to measure the contractions.[5] These measurements of contractility can be accompanied by determinations of intracellular $[Ca^{2+}]$, using fluorescent Ca^{2+}-indicators such as fura-2 or indo-1.[10] Isolated cardiomyocytes have proven to be especially valuable in studying the regulation of slow wave contractions in relation to SR function.[5]

1.1.4.   Assay of enzymes and isolation of intracellular organelles

Determinations of enzyme activities using broken cell preparations from whole hearts must take the cellular heterogeneity of the heart into consideration. For example, very little neutral cholesteryl esterase activity was detected in cardiomyocyte homogenates compared to whole ventricular extracts,[11] suggesting that the majority of neutral cholesteryl esterase activity in the heart is in nonmyocytic cells. Isolated cardiomyocytes also provide a useful experimental preparation to study the synthesis, processing, and degradation of enzymes and other proteins using pulse-time and pulse-chase experiments where the incorporation of [^{35}S]methionine into the enzyme/protein is measured. For example, in the adult heart, lipoprotein lipase is synthesized and processed by N-linked glycosylation in cardiomyocytes[12,13] before undergoing translocation to its functional binding site on the luminal surface of vascular endothelial cells.[14] The presence of specific proteins and evidence for gene expression in cardiomyocytes can also be detected by Western and Northern blotting, respectively. Immunohistochemical techniques can be utilized with permeabilized cardiomyocytes to investigate the subcellular localization of specific proteins.

  The isolation of membranes (e.g., sarcolemma) and organelles from cardiomyocytes also avoids potential contamination from nonmyocytic cells. Biochemical studies of SR membrane vesicles can be complemented by investigations of SR function in intact cardiomyocytes, by measuring caffeine-induced and rapid cooling-induced contractures.[10]

1.1.5. Receptors and signal transduction mechanisms

Isolated cardiomyocytes are well suited for radioligand binding studies so that receptors for drugs, hormones, and neurotransmitters can be localized to specific cell types in the heart. As a result, not only is the presence of specific receptors on cardiomyocytes documented, but quantitative information on receptor density (number of receptors per cell) and affinity for agonists and antagonists can be obtained.[15,16] Information from radioligand binding experiments complements functional analysis of receptor stimulation.[17] Xiao et al.[18] have recently reported that although both beta$_1$ and beta$_2$ adrenergic receptors coexist on cardiomyocytes, these receptor subtypes differ with respect to the signal transduction mechanisms used to produce specific cellular responses.

1.1.6. Pathophysiological studies

Incubation of hypoxic, substrate-deprived cardiomyocytes has been used as a model system for ischemic damage, where metabolic changes[19] as well as intracellular $[Ca^{2+}]$ measurements and contracture[20] can be monitored. The accumulation of intracellular metabolites in cardiomyocytes maintained in a static incubation under anoxic conditions may mimic the situation in ischemia where reduced perfusion will result in similar metabolic changes.

Cardiomyocytes isolated from experimental animals with diabetes and altered thyroid status retain the electrophysiological and metabolic changes that characterize whole heart or papillary muscle preparations,[7,21] thus establishing that at least some aspects of cardiac dysfunction in endocrine diseases reflect intrinsic changes in cardiomyocytes.

1.2. Limitations

Notwithstanding the extensive and effective use of isolated cardiomyocytes in the examples listed above, the question of whether studies with an isolated cell are truly representative of the situation in the intact heart must always be paramount in the mind of the investigator. It has been argued that short-term culture of isolated cardiomyocytes may be an important experimental approach,[22] so that the cells have time to "rest and repair" after the trauma of isolation procedures that involve exposure to low calcium concentrations and collagenase. Also, the preparation of cardiomyocytes from diseased hearts must be subject to the qualification that the isolated cells may not be representative because of selection bias for viable cells from the healthy portions of the myocardium.

1.3. History of Isolation Procedures

The historical development of cardiomyocyte isolation procedures has been described in a number of excellent reviews.[1,4,5,22,23] The chief problem to be overcome was the difficulty in isolating calcium-tolerant cardiomyocytes. Typically, hearts have to be perfused or incubated under nominally calcium-free conditions to loosen intercellular connections at intercalated discs.[1,5] The subsequent introduction of physiological concentrations of calcium often produced profound cellular damage (a form of calcium paradox). Thus, the principal technical advance over the last 15 years or so has been to develop isolation procedures that produce calcium-tolerant, quiescent cardiomyocytes. The procedure to be described for the isolation of cardiomyocytes from rat hearts was adapted from techniques published by Frangakis et al.[24] and Montini et al.,[25] with introduction of subsequent modifications based on more than 10 years of experience. [9,12,13,26-28]

2. Methodology for Isolating Cardiomyocytes

The isolation of cardiomyocytes involves two basic steps: (1) dissociation of myocytes from each other and from connective tissue by collagenase treatment at a low calcium concentration, and (2) selection of viable cardiomyocytes from damaged, nonviable myocytes and from nonmyocytic cells by low speed centrifugation and gravity sedimentation. A summary of the procedures is shown in Table 1.

TABLE 1

Summary of Procedures for Isolating Cardiomyocytes from Rat Hearts

1. Heart perfusion

    a. Heparinize rat (30–60 min)

    b. Remove heart and cannulate aorta for retrograde (Langendorff) perfusion with:

        i. MEM containing no added Ca^{2+} (4–5 min)

        ii. low-Ca^{2+} (25 μM) MEM containing collagenase (15 min)

    c. Remove ventricular tissue

2. Isolation of cardiomyocytes

    a. Wash ventricular tissue with low-Ca^{2+} MEM to remove any dead or damaged cells

    b. Incubate ventricular tissue with collagenase (in low-Ca^{2+} MEM) for approx. 7 min at 37°C in a shaking water bath

    c. Decant dislodged cells into a tube; wash undigested tissue twice and add released cells to the collagenase-released cells. Collect cells by low-speed (45 × g) centrifugation

    d. Resuspend cells into MEM containing 250 μM Ca^{2+}, centrifuge, and resuspend into MEM containing 500 μM Ca^{2+}

    e. Filter cells, and allow cardiomyocytes to settle at 1 × g (gravity sedimentation) for 15 min

    f. Resuspend cardiomyocytes into MEM containing 1 mM Ca^{2+}

    g. Determine cell yield and viability (percentage of rod-shaped cardiomyocytes that exclude Trypan blue) by microscopic examination.

2.1. Preparation of Solutions

Solution A

1. Add 1 liter of Millipore-purified water (>10 megohms resistivity) to one package of Joklik minimal essential medium (Gibco BRL Life Technologies, Burlington, ON; cat. no. 22300-016).
2. Then add 2 g $NaHCO_3$, 144 mg $MgSO_4$ (final concentration of 1.2 mM), and 198 mg DL-carnitine (final concentration of 1 mM).
3. Mix thoroughly and gas with 95% O_2: 5% CO_2.
4. After 30 min, adjust the pH to 7.4 with a few drops of 5 N NaOH.

Note: *Solution A is nominally Ca^{2+}-free, since no $CaCl_2$ is added.*

Solution B

1. Add 55 mg collagenase (Worthington Type II, 142 U/mg; Technicon Canada, Richmond, BC) and 100 mg essentially fatty acid-free bovine albumin (Sigma Chem. Co., St. Louis, MO; catalog no. A-6003) to 100 ml of solution A to give final concentrations of 78 mU/ml and 1 mg/ml (0.1% w/v), respectively.
2. Add 25 μl of 0.1 M $CaCl_2$ (final concentration of 25 μM). This quantity of solution B is sufficient for perfusion of one rat heart; 200 ml is prepared when two hearts are perfused.

Solution C

1. Add 1.25 g fatty acid-free bovine albumin to 125 ml solution A (final albumin concentration of 1% w/v). Various amounts of $CaCl_2$ are added sequentially to this solution during the isolation procedure to give final concentrations of 25 μM, 250 μM, 500 μM and 1 mM.

All solutions are maintained at 37°C in a shaking water bath, under an atmosphere of 95% O_2: 5% CO_2. Joklik MEM is convenient because the solid powder that is purchased is calcium free, so solutions with a range of calcium concentrations can be prepared. Also, the presence of the phenol red indicator allows for visual verification of proper pH control. The Joklik medium is supplemented with 1.2 mM $MgSO_4$ to enhance viability[25] and with carnitine to ensure adequate rates of fatty acid oxidation. A substantial portion of cardiac carnitine is lost during the isolation protocol.[5] Addition of taurine[8] has not improved either yield or viability of cardiomyocytes in our experience.

2.2.   Heart Perfusion

A male, Sprague-Dawley rat (200 to 250 g) is anesthetized with sodium pentobarbital (60 mg/kg body wt., i.p.). Heparin (Hepalean, from Organon Teknika, Toronto, ON; 2 U/g body wt. i.p.) is administered to the sedated rat 15 to 60 min prior to sacrifice by decapitation. After opening the chest, the heart is pulled upwards so that it can be excised with a scissor angled 45° to the body in such a way that a section of aorta is attached (at least 4 mm), and placed in solution A. Extraneous tissue (portions of lung and diaphragm) is removed to expose the aorta; the aortic arch and some of its branches are visible. The aorta is slipped over a cannula using two pairs of fine forceps and held in place with a crocodile or bulldog clamp for retrograde (Langendorff) perfusion with solution A for 4 min at room temperature to remove blood from the coronary circulation. During this initial perfusion, the heart is secured to the cannula with a 5-0 or 3-0 silk ligature, and extraneous tissue is removed.

The heart is then perfused with the collagenase-containing solution B (25 μM $CaCl_2$) at a flow rate of 6 to 7 ml/min (regulated by a Gilson Minipuls perfusion pump) at 37°C. The perfusion solution is not recirculated. After 5 min, the perfusate is collected for subsequent incubations. By perfusing with 100 ml solution B in a single-pass mode, the total perfusion time is 15 min or less. The heart becomes enlarged during this perfusion, with a light-brown appearance. During the perfusion with collagenase, the heart is gently "squeezed" between the thumb and index finger to monitor the dissociation; the heart should feel "soft" as opposed to hard (under-digested) or mushy (over-digested). Ventricular tissue is removed from the perfusion apparatus by cutting the cannulated heart below the atria with scissors, placed in a weigh boat containing solution C with 25 μM $CaCl_2$, and cut (teased) into 2 to 3 pieces.

Heparinization of the rat facilitates perfusion of the heart with solution A and the collagenase-containing solution B. Poorly perfused areas of the heart because of blood clots in the coronary vasculature are evident as dark-colored tissue with a harder texture when the ventricles are removed from the perfusion apparatus, and can be removed by dissection. It is also very important to ensure that no air bubbles are introduced into the system when the heart perfusion is changed from solution A to the collagenase-containing solution B.

The perfusion apparatus used in Calgary was purchased from the Apparatus Shop at Vanderbilt University, Nashville, Tennessee. This apparatus was originally designed for liver perfusions and the isolation of hepatocytes. Solution B is equilibrated by diffusion with 95% O_2:5% CO_2 in a rotating drum, so that gas exchange for oxygenation and pH control (CO_2:HCO_3- buffer) does not involve directly bubbling the gas mixture through this solution which contains both albumin and collagenase. The drums, perfusion pump, tubing, and bubble traps are all enclosed in a Plexiglas box maintained at 38°C. Cannulas were constructed from 13-gauge hypodermic stainless steel tubing. A groove (2 mm in length, 1/4 mm deep) in the cannula 2 mm from the end facilitates attachment of the aorta so that the aortic valve is not damaged. Two cannulas are inserted into a plastic holder, so our perfusion apparatus permits the perfusion of either one or two hearts. For two hearts, the volume of solution B is doubled and the Minipuls pump setting is adjusted to maintain flow rates of 6 to 7 ml/min. A two-heart procedure is utilized when a greater number of cardiomyocytes are required for study, or when cardiomyocytes are isolated from a control and experimental (e.g., diabetic) rat heart.[27]

A simpler and cheaper perfusion apparatus can be constructed easily; the components of the apparatus used in Vancouver are shown in Figure 1. A Cole Palmer motor and Masterflux speed controller make up the perfusion pump. Temperature is maintained at 37°C with a Haake circulating water pump. A lower bath is placed below the heart so that the perfusate can be recirculated in a closed system. The collagenase solution is bubbled with 95% O_2: 5% CO_2 using very fine tubing to keep foaming (of the albumin) to a minimum.

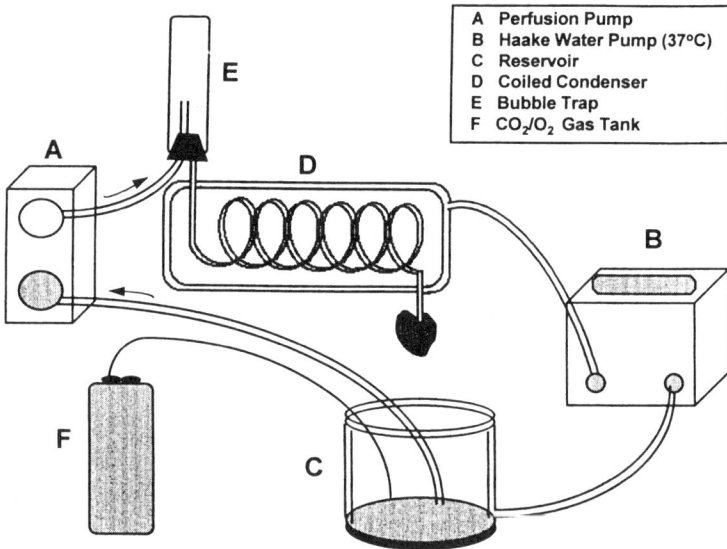

Figure 1
Perfusion apparatus for isolation of cardiomyocytes.

2.3. Isolation of Cardiomyocytes

Ventricular pieces in solution C containing 25 μM $CaCl_2$ are transferred to a 50 ml Erlenmeyer flask and incubated for 10 min at 37°C in a shaking water bath under an atmosphere of 95% O_2: 5% CO_2. The flask is then gently swirled and the medium (containing damaged and dead cells) is removed by aspiration. Solution B (13 ml of the perfusate collected from the heart perfusion) is added to the ventricular pieces and the incubation is continued at 37°C in the shaking water bath; the flask is occasionally shaken vigorously by hand to dislodge cells from the tissue pieces by mechanical agitation. After approximately 7 min, dissociated myocytes are decanted into a 50-ml plastic centrifuge tube. Residual (undigested) tissue pieces remaining in the flask are washed twice with 10 ml solution C containing 250 μM $CaCl_2$, and any additional dislodged cells are decanted into the same centrifuge tube containing myocytes dissociated into the collagenase-containing solution B. Some large tissue pieces may remain, particularly if the initial heart perfusion was poor. The digestion step with another 13 ml of solution B can be repeated a second time, but the viability of released cells tends to be low.

Cardiomyocytes in the centrifuge tube are collected by centrifugation (room temperature) at approximately $45 \times g$ for 0.5 to 1.5 min. The supernatant is removed carefully by aspiration, and the cell pellet is resuspended gently into 10 ml of solution C containing 250 μM $CaCl_2$. After centrifugation as before, the cells are resuspended in 15 ml of solution C containing 500 μM $CaCl_2$ and filtered through a 200-μm mesh silk screen to remove fine tissue debris. The cell suspension is finally allowed to settle for 15 min at $1 \times g$ (gravity sedimentation) under 95% O_2: 5% CO_2 at 37°C; viable, rod-shaped myocytes are larger and asymmetric (approximately 20×100 μm^1) and therefore settle more quickly than nonviable myocytes and other lighter cell types. Thus, sedimentation (low-speed centrifugation and gravity) is utilized to select for viable cardiomyocytes during the isolation procedure. After settling, the supernatant is removed carefully by aspiration, and the cardiomycytes are finally resuspended into 10 ml solution C containing 1 mM $CaCl_2$.

The step-wise exposure of the isolated cardiomyocytes to increasing $CaCl_2$ concentrations (from 25 μM to 250 μM to 500 μM) increases the percentage of cells that are viable (calcium tolerant) in 1 mM $CaCl_2$. The speed of centrifugation for the initial collection of cardiomyocytes is critical. Too low a speed may not remove the collagenase introduced into the medium from solution B; residual collagenase does not reduce viability but may influence cardiomyocyte function in subsequent incubations. On the other hand, centrifugation speeds that are greater than $45 \times g$ produce a densely packed pellet; as a result, cells are hypoxic and difficult to resuspend, and so cell viability is reduced. Similarly, a centrifuge tube with a large surface area to volume ratio must be used when cardiomyocytes are subjected to gravity $(1 \times g)$ sedimentation under an O_2 atmosphere in order to avoid hypoxia and loss of viability.

2.4. Determination of Yield and Viability

The yield of cardiomyocytes and viability is measured routinely by microscopic examination (Figure 2). An aliquot (20 μl) of the final cardiomyocyte suspension is mixed with an equal volume of 0.4% Trypan blue (in 0.9% NaCl) in a small plastic culture tube. After thorough mixing, cell number (9-μl aliquot) is determined microscopically using an improved Neubauer

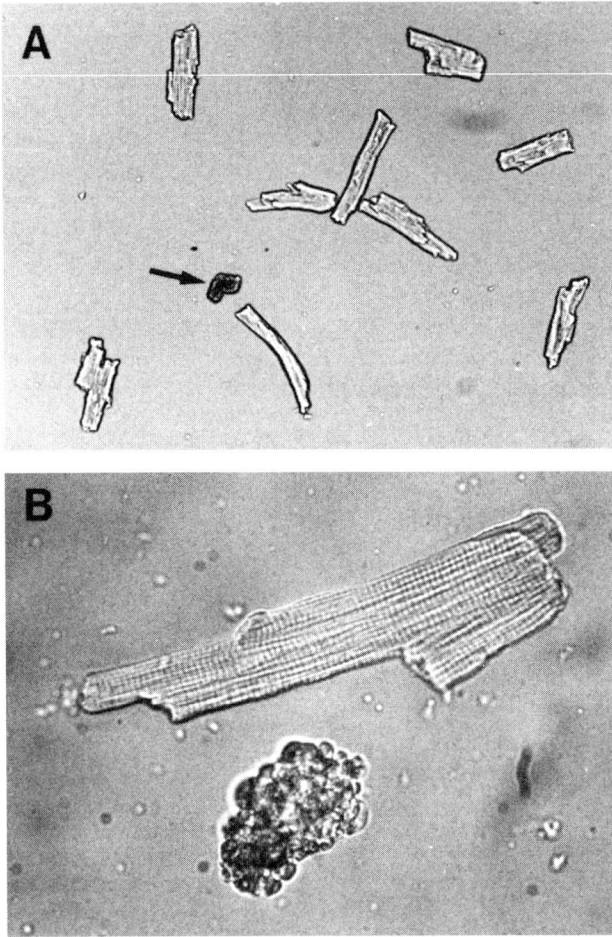

Figure 2

Panel **A** is a low power light micrograph of cardiomyocytes isolated from a rat heart. Viable cardiomyocytes are elongated, cylindrical cells; irregular shapes illustrate cleavage sites at branch points for intercellular connections (intercalated discs). The dark, round cell (arrow) is a Ca^{2+}-intolerant, nonviable myocyte that has taken up Trypan blue. Some viable cells have shortened (hypercontracted), presumably due to Ca^{2+} overload that precedes damage to sarcolemmal integrity. At higher magnification (panel **B**), clear separation at the intercalated disc region is apparent. Cross-striations (alternating light and dark transverse banding) are evident in the rod-shaped (approximate dimensions of 20×100 μm) viable cell. In comparison, the nonviable myocyte has a granular appearance. The cylindrical shape of cardiomyocytes is very evident with scanning electron microscopy; T-tubule openings can be observed on the cell surface. An intact glycocalyx and plasma membrane, abundant mitochondria, and well-defined myofibrils and Z bands are characteristic features of isolated cardiomyocytes examined by transmission electron microscopy (A.J. Kryski and D.L. Severson, unpublished observations).

hemocytometer. Total cell number is determined by counting all the cells in two sets of 16 squares. Viable cardiomyocytes are then counted, defined as those cells which are rod-shaped (20×100 μm) with clear cross-striations (alternating light and dark transverse binding) that exclude Trypan blue (Figure 2, panels A and B). Percentage viability is then calculated as viable cells/total cells × 100. On average, a single rat heart yields 12 to 14 × 10⁶ cells, with a viability of 80 to 85%.

Other more specialized tests of viability may be utilized, depending on the experimental use of the cardiomyocytes. Values for ATP and creatine phosphate content for our cardiomyocytes (22.3 ± 1.7 and 44.9 ± 7.0 µmol/g. dry wt. (n = 5), respectively) are somewhat higher, in fact, than levels reported for intact cardiac muscle.[5] Since the crude collagenase preparation used in the isolation procedure is contaminated with proteases, we have placed particular emphasis on demonstrating that the cell surface (plasma membrane) of the cardiomyocytes has not been altered substantially during the isolation process. A resting membrane potential of -71 mV ± 0.7 (n = 7) and an action potential configuration (e.g., amplitude of 81 ± 5 mV) that is consistent with recordings from intact cardiac tissue[4,5] indicate that sarcolemmal permeability and time- and voltage-dependent ion currents across the sarcolemma of cardiomyocytes are largely unchanged. Functional hormone receptors are also present on the surface of our isolated cardiomyocytes. For example, insulin receptors can be detected by radioligand binding (A.J. Kryski and D.L. Severson, unpublished observations) and by stimulatory effects of insulin on glucose oxidation[21,27] and protein synthesis.[27] Also, incubating cardiomyocytes with isoproterenol results in cyclic AMP accumulation[9] and activation of phosphorylase,[28] establishing the presence of functional beta-adrenergic receptors.

Biochemical studies typically require large numbers of cardiomyocytes, and so isolation procedures may have to emphasize yield over viability. By comparison, electrophysiological measurements on single cells allow the investigator to select only viable cells for study, so that neither yield nor viability is so critical.

Our results from biochemical studies of cardiomyocytes are typically reported on the basis of cell number. For example, lipoprotein lipase activity in cardiomyocyte homogenates ranges from 2 to 4 µmol oleate release per hour per 10⁶ cells.[26-28] Since cardiomyocytes are usually incubated in solution C which contains 1% (w/v) albumin (10 mg/ml), protein determinations are not a reliable method of normalizing for cell content unless the cells are washed extensively. An aliquot of the final cell suspension can also be added to a preweighed scintillation vial. After placing in an oven for at least 5 h, the dry weight of cells can be determined (typically 4.7 mg dry weight/10⁶ cells).[9] Using a wet-to-dry weight ratio of 4.35,[23] then the overall recovery of cardiomyoctyes is approximately 50% of the original heart (ventricular) wet weight.

2.5. Potential Problems

Two problems are likely to be encountered by an investigator who is attempting to isolate cardiomyocytes for the first time: poor digestion of the heart and low viability of isolated cardiomyocytes.

2.5.1. Poor dissociation of hearts

Two factors are critical for good dissociation of the heart. First, perfusion conditions are very important. The excised heart must be cannulated carefully, so as not to interfere with closure of the aortic valve; a substantial portion of the aorta must be attached to the heart for proper cannulation and perfusion. Prior heparinization of the rat greatly facilitates adequate perfusion of the isolated heart. Coronary flow must be controlled, and the pH, temperature and oxygenation status of the perfusion solution must be monitored.

The second factor is the source of collagenase. All collagenase (Worthington type II) preparations are partially purified from a bacterial source (*Clostridium histolyticum*), and thus contain contaminating protease activates (caseinase, trypsin, clostripain, and others). In fact, some degree of protease contamination is essential for dissociation of hearts.[5] Since the amount of protease contamination is variable in collagenase preparations, different lot numbers must be tested for effectiveness. This screening procedure can usually be conducted with small amounts (<1 g) of the individual lot numbers. Specific activities of different collagenase preparations vary greatly, and effective collagenase concentrations can range from 78 mU/ml to 429 U/ml. In general, the quicker the digestion time, the higher the yield of viable cells. Once an effective preparation has been identified, large quantities of the collagenase lot should be purchased (up to 100 g). Collagenase is supplied as a lyophilized powder, and is stable when stored in divided portions at $-80°C$; we have used a single collagenase preparation for more than 5 years. The intention to purchase bulk quantities of collagenase means that we only screen lot numbers where large quantities are available. Finally, bulk purchase has the economic advantage of allowing a reduced cost to be negotiated with the commercial supplier.

2.5.2. Low viability of isolated cardiomyocytes

The screen of collagenase preparations as mentioned above uses the yield of viable cardiomyocytes as one of the criteria of effectiveness, along with the extent of heart dissociation. Over-digestion with collagenase (good yield of cells but low viability) is usually apparent during the heart perfusion with solution B; the heart is pale and very flaccid when the ventricles are removed from the perfusion apparatus. The perfusion time can be decreased or, more reasonably, the concentration of collagenase should be reduced.

Occasionally, viability of cardiomyocytes will suddenly fall, even when using a collagenase preparation that has been effective previously. This finding typically implies a need for a thorough cleaning of the perfusion apparatus, although the use of ethanol to clean perfusion tubing should be avoided. The quality of water used to make up solutions A, B, and C can also vary despite Millipore filtration, probably because of the presence of variable concentrations of contaminating calcium. Therefore, different sources of water should be tested. Finally, we find that the presence of albumin in the isolation solutions and in the final medium for incubation is essential for maintenance of viability.

The use of essentially fatty acid-free bovine albumin minimizes variable contaminants and so we do not routinely screen albumin lot numbers, but investigators should always note when different albumin sources are used to correlate with their measurements of yield and viability. The control of pH, temperature, and oxygenation status is important. Isolated cardiomyocytes should always be maintained at room temperature or greater. Storage of isolated cardiomyocytes at 4°C must be avoided; cooling the cells results in intracellular Na^+ accumulation, which is followed by Na^+/Ca^{2+} exchange and calcium overload leading to cell death.[29]

Acknowledgments

The studies described in this paper were supported by operating grants from the Medical Research Council of Canada (DLS) and the Heart and Stroke Foundation of British Columbia and the Yukon (BR). The financial support of the Canadian Diabetes Association in the form of a scholarship to B. Rodrigues is gratefully acknowledged. The authors would like to thank Sylvia Chan for skilled secretarial assistance.

References

1. Dow, J.W., Harding, N.G.L., and Powell, T., Isolated cardiac myocytes. I. Preparation of adult myocytes and their homology with the intact tissue, *Cardiovasc. Res.*, 15, 483, 1981.
2. Blanchette-Mackie, E.J., Masuno, H., Dwyer, N.K., Olivecrona, T., and Scow, R.O., Lipoprotein lipase in myocytes and capillary endothelium of heart: immunocytochemical study, *Am. J. Physiol.*, 256, E818, 1989.
3. Camps, L., Reina, M., Llobera, M., Vilaró, S., and Olivecrona, T., Lipoprotein lipase: cellular origin and functional distribution, *Am. J. Physiol.*, 258, C673, 1990.
4. Dow, J.W., Harding, N.G., and Powell, T., Isolated cardiac myocytes. II. Functional aspects of mature cells, *Cardiovasc. Res.*, 15, 549, 1981.
5. Stemmer, P., Wisler, P.L., and Watanabe, A.M., Isolated myocytes in experimental cardiology, in *The Heart and Cardiovascular System,* 2nd ed., Fozzard, H.A. et al., Eds., Raven Press, New York, 1992, chap. 17.
6. Han, X., Shimoni, Y., and Giles, W.R., An obligatory role for nitric oxide in autonomic control of mammalian heart rate, *J. Physiol.*, 476, 309, 1994.
7. Shimoni, Y., Severson, D., and Giles, W.R., Effects of thyroid status and diabetes on regional differences in potassium currents in rat ventricle, *J. Physiol.*, 488, 673, 1995.
8. Bihler, I., Prayag, R., and Sawh, P.C., Influence of cell isolation and incubation procedures on Ca^{2+} dependence of glucose transport in isolated cardiac myocytes, *Can. J. Cardiol.*, 3, 23, 1987.

9. Kryski, A., Jr., Kenno, K.A., and Severson, D.L., Stimulation of lipolysis in rat heart myocytes by isoproterenol, *Am. J. Physiol.*, 248, H208, 1985.
10. Zhen, Y., Tibbits, G.F., and McNeill, J.H., Cellular functions of diabetic cardiomyocytes: contractility, rapid-cooling contracture, and ryanodine binding, *Am. J. Physiol.*, 266, H2082, 1994.
11. Stam, H., Broekhoven-Schokker, S., Schoonderwoerd, K., and Hülsmann, W.C., Cholesteryl esterase activities in ventricles, isolated heart cells and aorta of the rat, *Lipids*, 22, 108, 1987.
12. Carroll, R., Liu, L., and Severson, D.L., Post-transcriptional mechanisms are responsible for the reduction in lipoprotein lipase activity in cardiomyocytes from diabetic rat hearts, *Biochem. J.*, 310, 67, 1995.
13. Carroll, R., Ben-Zeev, O., Doolittle, M.H., and Severson, D.L., Activation of lipoprotein lipase in cardiac myocytes by glycosylation requires trimming of glucose residues in the endoplasmic reticulum, *Biochem. J.*, 285, 693, 1992.
14. Braun, J.E.A. and Severson, D.L., Regulation of the synthesis, processing and translocation of lipoprotein lipase, *Biochem. J.*, 287, 337, 1992.
15. Buxton, I.L.O. and Brunton, L.L., Direct analysis of β-adrenergic receptor subtypes on intact adult ventricular myocytes of the rat, *Circ. Res.*, 56, 126, 1985.
16. Buxton, I.L.O. and Brunton, L.L., Characterization of hormone receptors on the adult cardiac myocyte, in *Biology of Isolated Adult Cardiac Myocytes*, Clark, W.A., Decker, R.S., and Borg, R.K., Eds., Elsevier Science, 1988, 90.
17. Xiao, R.-P. and Lakatta, E.G., β₁-Adrenoceptor stimulation and their β₂-adrenoceptor stimulation differ in their effects on contraction, cytosolic Ca^{2+}, and Ca^{2+} current in single rat ventricular cells, *Circ. Res.*, 73, 286, 1993.
18. Xiao, R.-P., Hohl, C., Altschuld, R., Jones, L., Livingston, B., Ziman, B., Tantini, B., and Lakatta, E.G., β₂-Adrenergic receptor-stimulated increase in cAMP in rat heart cells is not coupled to changes in Ca^{2+} dynamics, contractility, or phospholamban phosphorylation, *J. Biol. Chem.*, 269, 19151, 1994.
19. Myrmel, T., Forsdahl, K., and Larsen, T.S., Triacylglycerol metabolism in hypoxic, glucose-deprived rat cardiomyocytes, *J. Mol. Cell. Cardiol.*, 24, 855, 1992.
20. Allshire, A., Piper, H.M., Cutherbertson, K.S.R., and Cobbold, P.H., Cytosolic free Ca^{2+} in single rat heart cells during anoxia and reoxygenation, *Biochem. J.*, 244, 381, 1987.
21. Rodrigues, B., Cam, M.C., and McNeill, J.H., Myocardial substrate metabolism: implications for diabetic cardiomyopathy, *J. Mol. Cell. Cardiol.*, 27, 169, 1995.
22. Jacobson, S.L., Techniques for isolation and culture of adult cardiomyocytes, in *Isolated Adult Cardiomyocytes, vol. 1, Structure and Metabolism*, Piper, H.M. and Isenberg, G., Eds., CRC Press, Boca Raton, FL, 1989, chap. 2.
23. Farmer, B.B., Mancina, M., Williams, E.S., and Watanabe, A.M., Isolation of calcium tolerant myocytes from adult rat hearts: review of the literature and description of a method, *Life Sci.*, 33, 1, 1983.
24. Frangakis, C.J., Bahl, J.J., McDaniel, H., and Bressler, R., Tolerance to physiological calcium by isolated myocytes from the adult rat heart; an improved cellular preparation, *Life Sci.*, 27, 815, 1980.

25. Montini, J., Bagby, G.J., Burns, A.H., and Spitzer, J.J., Exogenous substrate utilization in Ca^{2+}-tolerant myocytes from adult rat hearts, *Am. J. Physiol.*, 240, H659, 1981.

26. Rodrigues, B., Spooner, M., and Severson, D.L., Free fatty acids do not release lipoprotein lipase from isolated cardiac myocytes or perfused hearts, *Am. J. Physiol.*, 262, E216, 1992.

27. Braun, J.E.A. and Severson, D.L., Lipoprotein lipase release from cardiac myocytes is increased by decavanadate but not insulin, *Am. J. Physiol.*, 262, E663, 1992.

28. Severson, D.L., Carroll, R., Kryski, A., Jr., and Ramírez, I., Short-term incubation of cardiac myocytes with isoprenaline has no effect on heparin-releasable or cellular lipoprotein lipase activity, *Biochem. J.*, 248, 289, 1987.

29. Altschuld, R., Gibb, L., Ansel, A., Hohl, C., Kruger, F.A., and Brierley, G.P., Calcium tolerance of isolated rat heart cells, *J. Mol. Cell. Cardiol.*, 12, 1383, 1980.

Index

A

Acid, 95, *see also* Sodium-hydrogen exchange
Acidic solutions, 22
Acridine orange, 85, *see also* Sodium-hydrogen exchange
Actin/myosin, 2
Acylphosphate, 67–70, *see also* Na$^+$-K$^+$ ATPase, measurement
Adenosine diphosphate (ADP), 50–51, *see also* Na$^+$-K$^+$ ATPase, measurement
Adenosine triphosphate (ATP)
  Na$^+$-Ca$^+$ exchange regulation, 34
  Na$^+$-K$^+$ pump activity, 46, 65, 68–70
  viability of isolated cardiomyocytes, 111
ADP, *see* Adenosine diphosphate
ß-Adrenergic receptor, 18
Agarose gel, 74, 75
Air bubbles, 6, 107, *see also* Cardiomyocytes; Sarcoplasmic reticulum
Alamethicin, 47, 48, *see also* Na$^+$-K$^+$ ATPase, measurement
Albers-Post model, 64
Alcohol, 48, *see also* Na$^+$-K$^+$ ATPase, measurement
Amiloride, 89, *see also* Sodium-hydrogen exchange
Animal models, 22, *see also* Individual entries
Arrhythmias, 57, *see also* Na$^+$-K$^+$ ATPase, measurement
Asolectin, 34–35, *see also* Na$^+$-Ca$^+$ exchange
Assay procedure, 86–87, *see also* Sodium-hydrogen exchange
ATP, *see* Adenosine triphosphate
Atria, 71, *see also* Na$^+$-K$^+$ ATPase, measurement

B

BCECF, *see* 2',7'-Bis(carboxyethyl)-5(6)-carboxyfluorescein
Beta-adreneric antagonists, 103, *see also* Cardiomyocytes
Biochemical studies, 111, *see also* Cardiomyocytes
Biotinylated antibody technique, 73, *see also* Na$^+$-K$^+$ ATPase, measurement
2',7'-Bis(carboxyethyl)-5(6)-carboxyfluorescein (BCECF), 92–98, *see also* Sodium-hydrogen exchange
Bovine serum albumin (BSA)
  cardiomyocyte isolation, 106, 112–113
  myocardial sarcolemma isolation, 24, 25
  Na$^+$-K$^+$ pump activity, 69
Bradford assay, 24–27, *see also* Myocardial sarcolemma
BSA, *see* Bovine serum albumin
Buffers, 85, 87, 88–89, *see also* Sodium-hydrogen exchange

C

Calcium
  cardiomyocytes, 105, 109, 112
  contraction/relaxation, 2, 18, 32
  Na$^+$-Ca$^+$ exchange, 34, 35–37
  sarcoplasmic reticulum transport, 2–3
Calcium-ATPase, 2, 9, 10, 11, 32, *see also* Sarcoplasmic reticulum

Calcium oxalate, 11, *see also* Sarcoplasmic reticulum

Calcium pump, *see* Calcium-ATPase

Calcium release channel/ryanodine receptor, 2, 4, *see also* Sarcoplasmic reticulum

Calculations
myocardial sarcolemma isolation, 26–27, 28
Na^+-Ca^+ exchange measurement, 40–41

Calibration, 93, 96, 97, *see also* Sodium-hydrogen exchange

Calnexin, 3

Calsequestrin, 2, 3, 9–10, *see also* Sarcoplasmic reticulum

Cannulas, 107–108, *see also* Cardiomyocytes

Cardiac function, 18, 102, *see also* Cardiomyocytes; Myocardial sarcolemma

Cardiac glycosides, 55–57, 64, *see also* Na^+-K^+ ATPase, measurement; Ouabain

Cardiac sarcoplasmic reticulum, *see* Sarcoplasmic reticulum

Cardiomyocytes
history of isolation procedures, 104–105
limitations of preparations, 104
measurement of sodium-hydrogen exchange, 91–98
methodology for isolation, 105–113
myocardial sarcolemma isolation, 21
uses of isolated, 102–104

Cardiomyopathy, 3, *see also* Calcium

Carnitine, 106, *see also* Cardiomyocytes

Centrifugation
cardiac sarcoplasmic reticulum isolation, 5–8
low-speed and cardiomyocyte isolation, 105, 109
myocardial sarcolemma isolation, 18, 20, 22–23
Na^+-K^+ ATPase measurement, 48, 50

CHES buffer, 86, 87, *see also* Sodium-hydrogen exchange

Chick, 66, *see also* Na^+-K^+ ATPase, measurement

Cholestryl esterase, 103, *see also* Cardiomyocytes

Cleaning, 112, *see also* Cardiomyocytes

Clostridium histolyticum, 112, *see also* Cardiomyocytes

Collagenase, 105, 106, 107, 109, 111, 112, *see also* Cardiomyocytes

Compartmentation, 97, *see also* Sodium-hydrogen exchange

Computer
myocardial sarcolemma isolation, 26–27, 28
Na^+-Ca^+ exchange measurement, 40–41

Contamination
cardiomyocyte isolation, 112
myocardial sarcolemma isolation, 21
sarcoplasmic reticulum isolation, 9, 11
sodium-hydrogen exchange, 85

Contractility, 2–3, 18, 103, *see also* Calcium; Cardiomyocytes

Coupled enzyme assays, 51–53, *see also* Na^+-K^+ ATPase, measurement

Creatine phosphate, 111, *see also* Cardiomyocytes

Cross-contamination, 6, 19, *see also* Contamination; Sarcoplasmic reticulum; Myocardial sarcolemma

Cultured cell monolayers, 67, *see also* Na^+-K^+ ATPase, measurement

D

Densitometry, 73, 77, *see also* Na^+-K^+ ATPase, measurement

Density augmentation, 11

Density gradient centrifugation, *see also* Centrifugation
cardiac sarcoplasmic reticulum, 4, 6
myocardial sarcolemma isolation, 18, 20, 22–23

Deoxycholate (DOC), 47–49, *see also* Na^+-K^+ ATPase, measurement

DEPC, *see* Diethyl pyrocarbonate

Detergents, 47–49, *see also* Na^+-K^+ ATPase, measurement

Detergent-to-protein ratio, 48, *see also* Na^+-K^+ ATPase, measurement

Diabetes, 104, *see also* Cardiomyocytes

Diabetic cardiomyopathy, 84, *see also* Sodium-hydrogen exchange

Diethyl pyrocarbonate (DEPC), 74

Differential centrifugation, 4, 6–7, 18, 22–23, *see also* Centrifugation; Sarcoplasmic reticulum; Myocardial sarcolemma

Digitalis, 55, *see also* Cardiac glycosides; Na^+-K^+ ATPase, measurement

Digitoxigenin, 47, *see also* Na^+-K^+ ATPase, measurement

Dimethyl sulfoxide (DMSO), 51, *see also* Na^+-K^+ ATPase, measurement

Discontinuous sucrose density centrifugation, 6–8, 23, *see also* Centrifugation;

Sarcoplasmic reticulum;
Myocardial sarcolemma
Dissociation, 112, *see also* Cardiomyocytes
DMSO, *see* Dimethyl sulfoxide
DNase, 23
DOC, *see* Deoxycholate
Dog, 4, *see also* Sarcoplasmic reticulum
Drugs, 57, *see also* Na$^+$-K$^+$ ATPase,
measurement
Dyad junction, 2, *see also* Sarcoplasmic
reticulum
Dye loading, 91–98, *see also* Sodium-
hydrogen exchange

E

ECL, *see* Enhanced chemiluminescence
EGTA buffers, 33, 39, 40, 49, 51, *see also*
Na$^+$-K$^+$ ATPase, measurement;
Na$^+$-Ca$^+$ exchange
Electrophysiology, 4, 32, 102, *see also*
Cardiomyocytes; Na$^+$-Ca$^+$
exchange; Sarcoplasmic reticulum
Endocrine studies, 104, *see also*
Cardiomyocytes
Enhanced chemiluminescence (ECL)
technique, 73, *see also* Na$^+$-K$^+$
ATPase, measurement
Equilibrium studies, 65, 70, *see also* Na$^+$-K$^+$
ATPase, measurement
Excitation/contraction, 32, 46, *see also* Na$^+$-
K$^+$ ATPase, measurement; Na$^+$-
Ca$^+$ exchange
FKBP12.6, 3, *see also* Sarcoplasmic
reticulum

F

Fluorescence spectroscopy, 91–98, *see also*
Sodium-hydrogen exchange
Fluorescent markers, 85, *see also* Sodium-
hydrogen exchange
Fluorometric analysis, 54–55
Front door/back door phosphorylation, 67–70,
see also Na$^+$-K$^+$ ATPase,
measurement

G

Gel electrophoresis, 74, 75–76
Giant excised patch procedure, 32–33, *see
also* Na$^+$-Ca$^+$ exchange
Glucose, 102, *see also* Cardiomyocytes
Glucose-regulated protein (GRP94), 3, *see
also* Sarcoplasmic reticulum

Glycerol, 51, *see also* Na$^+$-K$^+$ ATPase,
measurement
Gradient fractionation, 23–24, *see also*
Myocardial sarcolemma
Gravity sedimentation, 105, 109, *see also*
Cardiomyocytes
GRP94, *see* Glucose-regulated protein 94
Guanidium thiocyanate-phenol-chloroform,
73–77

H

Heparinization, 107, 112, *see also*
Cardiomyocytes
HEPES buffer, 21, 66, 69, 87, *see also*
Buffers; Myocardial sarcolemma;
Na$^+$-K$^+$ ATPase, measurement;
Sodium-hydrogen exchange
Histidine buffer, 51, *see also* Na$^+$-K$^+$ ATPase,
measurement
Homogenization
myocardial sarcolemma isolation, 20,
21–22
sarcoplasmic reticulum, 4, 6, 7, 10–11
Horseradish peroxidase (HRP), 73, *see also*
Na$^+$-K$^+$ ATPase, measurement
HRP, *see* Horseradish peroxidase
Hypertension, 71, *see also* Na$^+$-K$^+$ ATPase,
measurement
Hypertrophy, 71, *see also* Na$^+$-K$^+$ ATPase,
measurement

I

Imidazole buffer, 51, *see also* Na$^+$-K$^+$
ATPase, measurement
Immunoblotting, 72, *see also* Na$^+$-K$^+$
ATPase, measurement
In vitro measurement, 34, *see also* Na$^+$-Ca$^+$
exchange
Initial rates, 38, *see also* Na$^+$-Ca$^+$
exchange
Inorganic phosphate, 49, 50, *see also* Na$^+$-K$^+$
ATPase, measurement
Inotropic drugs, 57–58, *see also* Na$^+$-K$^+$
ATPase, measurement
Insulin receptors, 111, *see also*
Cardiomyocytes
Intact cells, 65–67, *see also* Na$^+$-K$^+$ ATPase,
measurement
Interference, 67, *see also* Na$^+$-K$^+$ ATPase,
measurement
Ion channels, 2, 18, 102, *see also*
Cardiomyocytes; Myocardial
sarcolemma

Ischemia, 84, 104, *see also* Cardiomyocytes;
   Sodium-hydrogen exchange
Isobestic point, 93, 97, *see also* Sodium-
   hydrogen exchange
Isozymes, Na$^+$-K$^+$ pump, *see also* Na$^+$-K$^+$
   ATPase, measurement
   measurement overview, 70–71
   measurement using Northern blot, 73–77
   measurement using SDS-PAGE and
      Western blot, 72–73

K

K$_m$, 38, 40, *see also* Na$^+$-Ca$^+$ exchange
Kinases, 4, *see also* Sarcoplasmic
   reticulum

L

Lactate dehydrogenase (LDH), 51–53, *see
   also* Na$^+$-K$^+$ ATPase,
   measurement
Laemmli gel, 69, 72, *see also* Na$^+$-K$^+$
   ATPase, measurement
Landendorff heart, 107, *see also*
   Cardiomyocytes
LDH, *see* Lactate dehydrogenase
Leakiness, 33, 38, 47, 56–57, *see also* Na$^+$-
   Ca$^+$ exchange; Na$^+$-K$^+$ ATPase,
   measurement
Ligand binding, 19, *see also* Myocardial
   sarcolemma
LIGAND software, 56, *see also* Na$^+$-K$^+$
   ATPase, measurement; Ouabain
Limitations, 104, *see also* Cardiomyocytes
Lipid bilayer, 34–35, *see also* Na$^+$-Ca$^+$
   exchange
Lipolysis, 102–103, *see also* Cardiomyocytes
Lipoprotein lipase, 111, *see also*
   Cardiomyocytes
Liquid scintillation technique
   cardiac sarcoplasmic reticulum, 3, 9
   Na$^+$-Ca$^+$ exchange measurement, 37
   Na$^+$-K$^+$ pump activity, 67, 68
   sodium-hydrogen exchange, 86, 87

M

Magnesium ions, 55, *see also* Na$^+$-K$^+$
   ATPase, measurement; Mg$^+$-
   ATPase; Ouabain
Marker enzymes
   cardiac sarcoplasmic reticulum, 9
   myocardial sarcolemma isolation, 20,
      24–27, 46

Membrane potential, 35, *see also* Na$^+$-Ca$^+$
   exchange
Messenger ribonucleic acid (mRNA), 73–77,
   see also Na$^+$-K$^+$ ATPase,
   measurement
Metabolism, 102–103, *see also*
   Cardiomyocytes
Methionine, 103, *see also* Cardiomyocytes
3-*O*-Methyl fluorescein phosphate (MFP),
   54–55
MFP, *see* 3-*O*-Methyl fluorescein phosphate
Mg$^+$-ATPase, 46, 47, 52, *see also* Na$^+$-K$^+$
   ATPase, measurement
Mitochondria, 51, *see also* Contamination;
   Na$^+$-K$^+$ ATPase, measurement
MOPS, *see* 3-[*N*-Morpholino]-propane
   sulfonic acid
3-[*N*-Morpholino]propanesulfonic acid
   (MOPS) buffer, 21, 74
Myocardial sarcolemma
   contamination and cardiac sarcoplasmic
      reticulum isolation, 11
   history of isolation, 20
   isolation methodology, 20–27
   limitations of preparation, 19–20
   membrane vesicles, *see also* Vesicles
      function in isolated cardiomyocytes, 103
      sodium-hydrogen exchange, 85–91
   sedimentation rate, 4
   uses, 18–19
Myofiber, 2, 3
Myosin, *see* Actin/myosin

N

Na$^+$-Ca$^+$ exchange
   measurement
      history of procedures, 34
      limitations, 33–34
      methods, 32–33
      myocardial sarcolemma vesicles, 34–41
      proteins, 18, 19, 24
NADH, 51–53, *see also* Na$^+$-K$^+$ ATPase,
   measurement
Na$^+$-K$^+$ ATPase, measurement
   applications, 57
   assay, 49–51
   cardiac sarcoplasmic reticulum isolation, 9
   coupled enzyme assay, 51–53
   general considerations, 46–47
   membrane vesicles and detergent
      treatment, 47–49
   ouabain binding, 46, 55–57
   potassium-dependent phosphatase activity,
      53–55

Na$^+$-K$^+$ pump, 46, *see also* Na$^+$-K$^+$ ATPase, measurement

Nigericin, 96, *see also* Sodium-hydrogen exchange

Nitrophenylphosphatase, potassium-dependent, 24–27, 53–55, *see also* Marker enzymes; Myocardial sarcolemma; Na$^+$-K$^+$ ATPase, measurement

Nonlinear least squares analysis, 9, *see also* Sarcoplasmic reticulum

Nonspecific binding, 67, *see also* Na$^+$-K$^+$ ATPase, measurement; Rubidium

Northern blot analysis, 73–77, 103, *see also* Cardiomyocytes; Na$^+$-K$^+$ ATPase, measurement

O

Orientation, vesicles, 33, *see also* Myocardial sarcolemma; Na$^+$-Ca$^+$ exchange

Orthophosphorate, 69–70, *see also* Na$^+$-K$^+$ ATPase, measurement

Orthophosphoric acid (TAP), 68, *see also* Na$^+$-K$^+$ ATPase, measurement

Ouabain
  myocardial sarcolemma isolation, 25
  Na$^+$-K$^+$ ATPase
    binding, 55–57, 65–66, 67, 68–70
    measurement, 46, 47–50, 52, 54

Oxygenation, 98, 113, *see also* Cardiomyocytes

P

Passive efflux, 39–40, *see also* Na$^+$-Ca$^+$ exchange

Patch clamp technique, 102, *see also* Cardiomyocytes

Pathophysiological studies, 104, *see also* Cardiomyocytes

PEP, *see* Phosphoenolpyruvate

Permeability, 38, 85, *see also* Na$^+$-Ca$^+$ exchange; Sodium-hydrogen exchange

pH
  cardiomyocyte isolation, 106, 113
  myocardial sarcolemma isolation, 21–22
  Na$^+$-K$^+$ ATPase measurement, 50
  sodium-hydrogen exchange, 84, 89, 93–95

Phosphatase, potassium-dependent, 53–55

Phosphoenolpyruvate (PEP), 51–53, *see also* Na$^+$-K$^+$ ATPase, measurement

Phosphoenzyme, 68–69, *see also* Na$^+$-K$^+$ ATPase, measurement

Phosphorylated intermediates, 67–70, *see also* Na$^+$-K$^+$ ATPase, measurement

Phosphorylation, 46

Photobleaching, 97–98, *see also* Sodium-hydrogen exchange

PI, *see* Purification index

Pig, 6–7, *see also* Sarcoplasmic reticulum

PK, *see* Pyruvate kinase

Polyclonal antibodies, 71, *see also* Na$^+$-K$^+$ ATPase, measurement

Polyvinylidene difluoride (PVDF) membrane, 72, *see also* Na$^+$-K$^+$ ATPase, measurement

Potassium chloride
  myocardial sarcolemma isolation, 22
  Na$^+$-Ca$^+$ exchange measurement, 35, 36, 40
  sodium-hydrogen exchange, 89

Potassium ionophore, *see* Valinomycin

Potassium ions, 65, *see also* Na$^+$-K$^+$ ATPase, measurement; Ouabain

Protease, 112, *see also* Cardiomyocytes; Contamination

Proteins
  cardiomyocytes, 103
  myocardial sarcolemma isolation, 19
  Na$^+$-Ca$^+$ exchange measurement, 35
  Na$^+$-K$^+$ ATPase, 66

Proteoliposomes, 33, *see also* Na$^+$-Ca$^+$ exchange

Proteolytic inhibitors, 72, *see also* Na$^+$-K$^+$ ATPase, measurement

Purification, 24–27, *see also* Myocardial sarcolemma

Purification index (PI), 27, *see also* Myocardial sarcolemma

Purity, 8–9, *see also* Sarcoplasmic reticulum

PVDF, Polyvinylidene difluoride membrane

Pyruvate kinase (PK), 51–53, *see also* Na$^+$-K$^+$ ATPase, measurement

R

Radioisotopes
  Na$^+$-Ca$^+$ exchange measurement, 32
  sarcoplasmic reticulum isolation, 3, 8–9
  sodium-hydrogen exchange, 85, 86

Radioligand binding studies, 104, 111, *see also* Cardiomyocytes

Rapid uptake device (RUD), 38, 39, *see also* Na$^+$-Ca$^+$ exchange

Rat
  cardiomyocyte isolation, 102, 105–113
  isozymes of Na$^+$-K$^+$ pump, 71, *see also* Sodium pump

sodium-hydrogen exchange, 85–91
Receptors, 104, 111, *see also* Cardiomyocytes
Recovery, 19, 23, 24–27, *see also* Myocardial
    sarcolemma
Resting tension, 57, 98, 102, 111, *see also*
    Cardiomyocytes; Na+-K+ ATPase,
    measurement; Sodium-hydrogen
    exchange
Rubidium-86, 66–67, 70, *see also* Na+-K+
    ATPase, measurement
RUD, *see* Rapid uptake device
Ryanodine receptor, 3, 8–10, *see also*
    Sarcoplasmic reticulum

S

Sarcolemma, *see* Myocardial sarcolemma
Sarcoplasmic reticulum
    applications, 2–4
    centrifugation, 5–8
    data obtained, 9–10
    excitation-contraction coupling and
        calcium pump, 32
    potential problems, 10–11
    preparation of solutions, 5
    purity determination, 8–9
Scatchard plot, 56, 57, *see also* Na+-K+
    ATPase, measurement; Ouabain
Scintillation technique, *see* Liquid
    scintillation technique
SDS, *see* Sodium dodecyl sulfate
SDS-PAGE, *see* Sodium dodecyl sulfate
    polyacrylamide gel
    electrophoresis
Sedimentation rate, 4, *see also* Differential
    centrifugation; Sarcoplasmic
    reticulum
Sheep, 4, *see also* Sarcoplasmic reticulum
Signal transduction, 104, *see also*
    Cardiomyocytes
Signal-to-noise ratio, 19, 34, 35, *see also*
    Myocardial sarcolemma; Na+-Ca+
    exchange
Slow wave contractions, 103, *see also*
    Cardiomyocyte
SNARF-1, 92, *see also* Sodium-hydrogen
    exchange
Sodium, 65, *see also* Na+-K+ ATPase,
    measurement; Ouabain
Sodium chloride, 30, 35, 36, *see also* Na+-
    Ca+ exchange
Sodium-calcium exchange, *see* Na+-Ca+
    exchange
Sodium dodecyl sulfate polyacrylamide gel
    electrophoresis (SDS-PAGE)

Na+-K+ pump activity, 67, 68, 69, 70–73
sarcoplasmic reticulum isolation, 9
Sodium dodecyl sulfate (SDS), 47–49, 55,
    Na+-K+ ATPase, measurement;
    Ouabain
Sodium-hydrogen exchange
    cardiomyocytes, 91–98
    sarcolemmal membrane vesicles, 85–91
Sodium pentobarbital, 107, *see also*
    Cardiomyocytes
Sodium-potassium ATPase, *see* Na+-K+
    ATPase, measurement
Sodium pump
    intact cells, 65–67
    Na+-K+ ATPase isozymes, 70–77
    phosphorylated intermediates, 67–70
Sodium pyrophosphate, 22, *see also*
    Myocardial sarcolemma
Sodium transport, hydrogen-dependent, *see*
    Sodium-hydrogen exchange
Sodium/potassium ATPase, *see* Na+-K+
    ATPase, measurement
Solubilization, 47, *see also* Na+-K+ ATPase,
    measurement
Son of RUD, 38, 39, *see also* Na+-Ca+
    exchange
Sorcin, 3, *see also* Sarcoplasmic reticulum
Spectrofluorometer, 93, 94, *see also* Sodium-
    hydrogen exchange
Spectrophotometry, 57, *see also* Na+-K+
    ATPase, measurement; Ouabain
Spectroscopy, 25, *see also* Myocardial
    sarcolemma
Stop solutions, 89, *see also* Sodium-hydrogen
    exchange
Storage, 85, 113, *see also* Cardiomyocytes;
    Sodium-hydrogen exchange
Succinate dehydrogenase, 9, *see also*
    Sarcoplasmic reticulum
Sucrose density centrifugation
    myocardial sarcolemma isolation, 18, 20,
        22–23
    Na+-K+ ATPase measurement, 47, 51
    sarcoplasmic reticulum isolation, 6–8
    sodium-hydrogen exchange, 87

T

TAP, *see* Orthophosphoric acid
Taurine, 106, *see also* Cardiomyocytes
TBS bloto, 72, *see also* Na+-K+ ATPase,
    measurement
TBST buffer, 72, 73, *see also* Buffers; Na+-
    K+ ATPase, measurement
TCA, *see* Trichloroacetic acid

Temperature, regulation
  cardiomyocyte isolation, 113
  myocardial sarcolemma isolation, 21
  Na$^+$-K$^+$ ATPase measurement, 50, 69
  sarcoplasmic reticulum isolation, 5
  sodium-hydrogen exchange, 97
TES buffer, 21, *see also* Buffers; Myocardial
      sarcolemma
Thyroid status studies, 104, *see also*
      Cardiomyocytes
Time dependence, 38, *see also* Na$^+$-Ca$^+$
      exchange
Tissumizer, 22
Tracking dyes, 69, *see also* Na$^+$-K$^+$ ATPase,
      measurement
Translot cell, 72, *see also* Na$^+$-K$^+$ ATPase,
      measurement
Transmembrane potential, 64, *see also* Na$^+$-
      K$^+$ ATPase, measurement
Transport systems, 2, *see also* Calcium
Transverse tubules, 2, *see also* Sarcoplasmic
      reticulum
Trichloroacetic acid (TCA), 50, 67, 68, 69,
      see also Na$^+$-K$^+$ ATPase,
      measurement
Tris-HCl buffer, 48–50, 51, 55–56, 68, 69,
      see also Na$^+$-K$^+$ ATPase,
      measurement
Troponin C, 2
Trypan blue, 109–111, *see also*
      Cardiomyocytes

V

V_{max}, 38, 40, *see also* Na$^+$-Ca$^+$ exchange
Valinomycin, 35, 36, *see also* Na$^+$-Ca$^+$
      exchange

Vanadate, 46, 50, *see also* Na$^+$-K$^+$ ATPase,
      measurement
Vesicles, *see also* Myocardial sarcolemma
  detergent treatment, 47–49
  myocardial sarcolemma isolation,
      19–20
  Na$^+$-Ca$^+$ exchange measurement,
      34–41
  sarcoplasmic reticulum, 3, 4
Vesicular orientation, 47, *see also* Na$^+$-K$^+$
      ATPase, measurement
Vesicular volume, 33, 38, *see also* Na$^+$-Ca$^+$
      exchange
Viability, 109–111, 112–113, *see also*
      Cardiomyocytes
Voltage clamp technique, 34, 102, *see also*
      Cardiomyocytes; Na$^+$-Ca$^+$
      exchange

W

Western blot analysis, 10, 72–73, 103, *see also*
      Cardiomyocytes; Na$^+$-K$^+$ATPase,
      measurement; Sarcoplasmic
      reticulum

Y

Yield
  cardiomyocyte isolation, 109–111
  myocardial sarcolemma isolation,
      24–27

Z

Zeta-probe, 76–77, *see also* Na$^+$-K$^+$ ATPase,
      measurement